PLANT-BASED KETO

4 WEEKS KETOGENIC VEGAN MEAL PLAN TO LOSE WEIGHT, ENERGIZE YOUR BODY, IMPROVE YOUR SPORTS NUTRITION, MEAL PLANNING AND YOUR STRENGHT THANKS TO THIS PLANT BASED VEGAN KETO MEAL PLAN

Table of Contents

Introduction

There are so many diets in today's society that can be beneficial to our minds, bodies, and health. One of the most popular diets that people transition to is being a vegan. As with any diet you choose, you should consult your doctor and find out if it is safe for you. In this book, we're going to give you vital information about this diet to help give you more information as well. It may be for animal rights, the planet, or maybe they just want to get healthier. Some also have religious, moral, or ethical reasoning behind their decision to be vegan. There are many benefits to adopting this lifestyle but the first thing we need to understand is what is a vegan? A vegan is someone who does not eat or use animal products. This means you need to cut out a lot of things you take for granted such as milk, eggs, cheese, honey, butter and more. Of course, one of the obvious things about a vegan diet is no meat of any kind. You'll have to rethink your dairy, meal plans, even the makeup and clothes you wear or the shampoo you use for your hair. This means you will have to either keep them out altogether from your life or replace them with vegan-friendly options. With so many people turning toward veganism, it's been said that it's turned into a movement by many articles and even some news stations, companies are listening and making amazing new products that are vegan-friendly thereby making it easier than ever to adopt this lifestyle and reap the benefits.

There is really only one way to be a vegan as opposed to other diets where they have subsections and other variations. However, while the definition of being a vegan is solid, there are many different ways to exact a vegan diet. Many have pros and cons and it's up to you to determine which one is the best for your issues and health. It's also important to do your research because some of the diets that claim to be vegan are not because they add meat and dairy into the diet later on after the first few weeks. This is obviously not a vegan diet and therefore not recommended for the changes you're trying to make in your lifestyle.

Some of the most popular vegan diets that people have either been wanting to try or have been curious about are the 'raw till four diet' which has been made amazingly popular due to a vegan on a viral video site.

This book is about showing you what it means to be vegan as well as how you can lose weight naturally and quickly from a popular diet that seems to go against everything a vegan lifestyle entails. This diet is called the ketogenic diet. The ketogenic diet is a high-fat diet that promotes the reduction of carbohydrates so that the body can use energy in a more efficient and cleaner way. Even though this is a high-fat diet, it is very effective at helping the practitioner lose weight safely and naturally.

My hope is that you gain extreme value with every word that you read so that you can live a healthier and happier life while upholding ideals that will benefit not only the planet and animals but future generations as well.

Chapter 1: What is plant-based keto

The modern world is now well aware of the concept of a keto diet. And if anyone does not have the idea of a keto diet! It is a modernly designed diet plan which has restrictions. After following those restrictions, the person might obtain several benefits. A ketogenic diet plan allows you to take fewer carbs in a day. This means in the ketogenic diet plan you have to lower your carb intake. The story does not finish here.

Along with this, you have to increase your fat intake. Moderate your protein. So a ketogenic diet plan says to lower the carb intake and increase fat intake keeping the proteins moderate. It has been said and as well as proved to give us several benefits. Significant of them is weight loss. The food we eat is either derived from a plant source, or it is an animal product. In the keto meal plans, we have several, and plant foods and all of them are keto friendly. Limiting your food interest to that specified too items is the key to success in case of ketogenic diet plan.

Life is nothing without innovation. This is the era of advancements where each day brings us something admirable. Whenever a plan is made it does not stay the same forever and is altered. All of those alterations are good and are for the betterment of individuals. It is what Vegan Keto Diet brings us. It is a modern version of the ketogenic diet plan.

Vegan Keto diet as the name indicates there is a modernized version of the ketogenic diet. In this updated version focus is only on plant-derived food.

It means that we cannot eat the foods that are from the animal source. Though those products are keto friendly, this new version says us to eat only plant-based foods. If a person will eat a vegan diet that he will adapt according to the instructions of the vegan keto diet. He has to refrain or entirely separate from the animal foods and would have to restrict himself to plant-based foods. Though it is difficult to manage the carb intake while eating a vegan diet if we will give it required attention then is possible to stay at low carb she eating a vegan keto diet.

A ketogenic diet is a diet that is rich in fats low at carbs and moderate at proteins. The maximum limit if carb intake is 50g for a day. This means that the person cannot eat more than 50g if carbs while following a ketogenic diet plan. Reduction of carbs from this specified value helps the body to adopt a state in which it utilizes fats as a source of energy. It is called ketosis. During ketosis, a person burns fats rather than carbohydrates to prepare power for the body's metabolism. This tells us that those who would follow the ketogenic diet plan would consume fat mostly. And that fat is obtained from an animal source as 75% of your food intake would be fatty, so the person following a keto diet plan automatically eats animal-based foods. These are loaded with fats, for example, meat, butter, and full-fat dairy products.

Those people who are vegetarians can quickly adapt to a ketogenic diet or a vegan diet plan. Vegans can only eat plant-based foods like grains, vegetables, fruits, and other products which are prepared using a plant source. Vegans do not have to eat those food items which are based on the animal source. When a person follows a ketogenic diet plan, his body metabolism starts doing ketosis that is the utilization of fats for energy. From the previous sentence, the availability of lipids and their use during the usage of ketogenic can be understood. This diet plan demands to limit the carb intake as well. So to limit the carb intake and eat food full of fats the person following a ketogenic diet plan consumes animal products. This does not mean that then the person can't shift to ketosis in some other way. And yes we can do the same by using a vegan keto diet.

We should give our body the proper time to adjust itself with the plant-based foods. For a vegan keto eater, it is necessary to understand the importance of vegetables, fruits, and plant-based foods. We know that a vegan keto diet allows you to consume food that is obtained from a plant source. So following this diet plan, you have to give up all kinds of animal-based foods as the name "Vegan Keto" indicates! You have to alter the keto diet trend. Just omit the keto-friendly animal products and limit your food consumption to plant-based foods only. It is necessary for us to understand the importance and benefits of food items that are obtained from a plant source. Let's have a look at the numerous reasons which compel us to eat plant-based foods.

How to Get Started with the Keto Vegan Diet

There are two ways you can get started with a keto vegan diet. The first way is by simply jumping right in and cutting out all carbohydrates from your diet. This method can be quite shocking as the transition is very steep. However, the practitioner usually sees results in a quicker time frame and is less likely to deal with sugar withdrawal symptoms for a long period of time.

The second way involves slowly implementing keto vegan practices. This involves slowly reducing your carbohydrate consumption by progressively eating low amounts of carbs every day. The second way is less jarring to beginner practitioners and allows for a learning curve that is not so steep. While it can be easier for newbie keto vegan practitioners to follow the second method, it takes longer to see noticeable results.

The method that you choose to start the keto vegan diet is entirely up to you and depends on your goals and lifestyle. You can start by practicing one method, and then the other to see what works best for you.

No matter how you get started here are a few tips that are useful:

• Clear the non-keto vegan foods out of your cupboards and refrigerator and fill them up with keto-vegan friendly food so that you have an easier time sticking to this diet.

• Keep things simple at the beginning. Simply up your fat and protein intake and ensure that you are consuming less than 50 grams of carbohydrates every day without worrying too much about the comparative proportions of each. Adjust to the diet then worry about these later.

• Consult a licensed health care practitioner before you begin the keto vegan diet. Ensure that you do not have any preexisting medical conditions that might need addressing before you begin this diet.

Side Effects of the Keto Vegan Diet

Transitioning into a keto vegan lifestyle can be quite an adjustment and this has physical implications. It is not uncommon for new practitioners of the keto vegan diet to experience a condition known as the keto flu. Keto flu symptoms can include:

• Muscle cramps

• Low energy and weakness

• Dizziness

• Sleep disturbances

• Fatigue

• Poor concentration

• Diarrhea

• Constipation

• Nausea

• Headaches

• Irritability The keto flu is typically experienced by people who jump right into this diet and follow all the rules off the bat. People who allow themselves to ease into this diet and lifestyle are less likely to experience the keto flu as the body is trained to slowly start burning more and more fat as carbohydrates are slowly removed from the diet.

The keto flu is typically caused by the alteration in water and mineral balances that the ketogenic vegan diet causes. You can restore this balance, and thereby curb the side effects of the keto flu, by adding more salt to your diet and taking mineral supplements such as sodium, potassium, and magnesium. These supplements are especially great at easing headaches, insomnia and muscle aches.

Additional supplements and substances that can aid in fighting the side effects of the keto flu include:

• Exogenous ketones. These are simply ketones that are synthesized outside your body. Taking the supplement increases blood ketone levels and therefore, helps fight keto flu.

• MCT oil. As mentioned earlier, this oil skips the digestive process and goes directly to the liver to be converted into ketones. This allows less of an adjustment period for your body to develop higher levels of ketones and thus, fights the symptoms of the keto flu. You can simply drink this oil as is or add it to your smoothies and other dishes

• Caffeine. Low energy is a common symptom of the keto flu and caffeine helps fight this symptom by boosting energy. Caffeine also increases athletic performance, increases fat loss, and reduces the risk of developing type 2 diabetes. You can increase the supply of caffeine in your diet by consuming unsweetened coffee and tea.

Other strategies that can be implemented to fight keto flu include staying hydrated, eating fiber-rich foods, engaging in light activity, and getting adequate rest.

Luckily, the symptoms of the keto flu typically only last for a few days and the practitioner can continue with his or her life without any negative consequence.

Adjusting your Carbs while Being on Vegan Keto Diet

The rule of the vegan keto diet is to limit carbs and to stay away from animal-based food. But how would you do that? When a person is on a ketogenic diet, he can only consume 50g carbs per day. The modern vegan keto diet is more restricting. It asks you to eat only 30g of net carbs a day. After knowing this, we might feel confused because this isn't easy! Though the modern version of keto might fluctuate at carbs but still the net carb intake is deficient as compared to the value taken by an average person.

There are some rules which you have to follow to get maximum benefits. Firstly, isolate the food items that are high in carbs, and they include bread, pasta, wheat, and rice that we frequently eat. Fruits though delicious but are a rich source of sugars, and we know sugars are the carbs which aren't vegan keto friendly so do not go for fruits except the ones that are listed above. Otherwise, the results could be devastating. If we aren't eating fruits rich in carbs, then it's understood that we would refrain from high carb vegetables. Avoid the use of such sauces and dressings that have high sugar content. There is a trick that you can do when you desperately desire to eat something full of carbohydrates. For example, boiled and mashed cauliflower can replace potatoes. Zucchini can be grated to look like noodles.

If you have a workout as a part of your routine, then what would you do? Do not go for exercise in the starting two weeks when you begin with vegan keto diet plan and let your body adapt the new approach. When you start with vegan keto diet plan, you limit carbs that are the immediate source of energy. After this, your body has to work on fats by adopting ketosis, and this is indeed a big transition, and for adjusting with it, your body needs some time. This is the time during which you have to refrain from the workout. The other significant change is the shift of source of fats which were previously obtained from animal source but now would be obtained from a plant source. As the path is complicated to let your body adopt it steadily and do not opt for a workout in the beginning.

Acquire the required Amount of Proteins during Vegan Keto Diet

When you are following a different diet plan than your regular meals, then you have to put in particular focus. As on vegan keto diet, we have to eat a moderate amount of proteins so its necessary to keenly observe the intake. Your protein requirement is 0.7g per pound. This value could exceed 1. During vegan keto, only plant food is allowed to look for protein sources from plants. On average 100-200g is the protein required. Almonds and sunflower seeds are two good sources of proteins, but they give you carbs enough to disturb your schedule. Here hemp seeds are a good option. They offer 30g proteins and 8g fibers in half cup. Consume tofu and tempeh because they have enough proteins. Three ounces of seitan gives you 18g protein and a few carbs.

The people who exercise during vegan keto diet plan must fulfill their protein requirements by taking supplements. A rice-pea powder is available, and it is used as a protein supplement during exercise. Athletes who follow a ketogenic diet plan obtain abundant proteins from an animal source. The essential amino acids are responsible for their excellent health, and if athletes face there a shortage, protein deficiencies will result. It is not easy to fulfill the demand of those essential proteins by plant source so they must render a greater focus. Here one option could be to use a combination of foods to get maximum proteins. When different amino acids aggregate, they might give them complete proteins. This shows the significance of a diverse menu. A variety of plant-based protein sources is the solution for athletes to fulfill protein demand during the vegan keto diet plan.

Food Options to replace the Animal-Based Feed

During vegan keto, we can't eat anything that has been obtained by animals. So we need plant substitutes for all those food ingredients. This transition is not as simple as you think because you might switch to new options with intellect so that you may not harm yourself during this. Do not eat processed fats during vegan keto diet plan and check the food you are eating to make sure that the food is free if all kinds of unfriendly ingredients.

In the Case of Dairy Foods

• Replace milk with coconut milk and almond cream

• Coconut cream should replace the other cream

• Coconut oil should replace butter

• Flaxseed should replace eggs for cooking and eggs for meal shall be replaced by silken tofu and veggies In the case of grains and starches

• Replace pasta by shirataki noodles and zucchini

• Peanut butter pancakes can replace pancakes

• Cauliflower rice would be best for replacement of rice

• Chia pudding can replace cereals

• Lettuce wraps would replace sandwich bread

• Flax tortillas would replace tortillas Substitutes for snacks

• Dehydrated vegetables can replace chips and give you pleasure

• Chia seed crackers can replace crackers Substitutes for desserts

• Avocado pudding can replace pudding you eat normally

• Ice-cream can be replaced by avocado ice-cream

• Nuts could give you the deliciousness of brownies.

Processed soya beans are an excellent option to replace meat. They could give us some proteins. Protein powders are also available in the market. Soybeans must not be eaten in excess; otherwise they would harm you. Within certain limits, they would not be dangerous. It can affect the hormone testosterone which means it would harm men more if taken above description. We are fond of snacks, desserts, condiments, sauces and other additional food items to our meals that we can't think to give up those, so we surely need replacements. However, alternatives for staples like wheat and grains are crucial.

Chapter 2: Body cleansing

The Science Behind Ketosis and How it Aids in Weight Loss Management

The reason that the ketogenic diet is so efficient at not only causing weight loss but improving overall health is that it replaces carbohydrate intake with healthy fat intake. This shifts the body away from metabolizing carbohydrates and towards metabolizing fat in an effort to gain energy. Simply put, when you practice the ketogenic diet, your body no longer uses standard sugar to gain energy but instead burns body fat, which can lead to weight loss in addition to many more significant health benefits.

The ketogenic diet has been around for over 100 years and was initially developed in an effort to fight epilepsy. However, its many other health benefits and its efficiency at causing weight loss cannot be denied.

This diet causes weight loss through a process known as ketosis. Ketosis is a metabolic state that only occurs when foods that are rich in carbohydrates are restricted. This restriction forces the body to look for alternative fuel sources and it turns to fat for that source. Ketosis can occur naturally such as when a person is fasting, during pregnancy or during starvation. If you have ever skipped a meal or two or partook in strenuous exercise then you have likely undergone this process unknowingly. Practicing the ketogenic diet is a less extreme way of forcing the body to seek out alternative sources of energy.

The process is so named because the fat molecules transformed into an energy source are called ketones. Ketones are fat-derived energy molecules that are generated in the liver and flows through the bloodstream. When the term 'ketones' or 'ketone bodies' is used, it typically refers to three main types. The first two are called acetoacetate and beta-hydroxybutyrate. They are more abundant that the third type, which is called, acetone.

Ketones are always present in the blood, but their presence increases dramatically when there are conditions that force the body away from metabolizing carbohydrates. They are used by the major organs such as the brain, heart, and kidney. Ketosis and therefore, ketones are particularly important to the brain because the brain has no other way of deriving energy apart from the metabolism of carbohydrates and fats.

How Ketosis Occurs

Before the process of ketosis is activated, gluconeogenesis occurs. Gluconeogenesis is the process whereby used non-carbohydrate components like amino acids, which are the units from which proteins are made, produce energy. This process occurs when sugar intake is limited and glycogen, which is your body's storage of sugar is being used. As glycogen becomes depleted, gluconeogenesis increases and jumpstarts the fat burning process even though ketone production does not yet occur at this point.

The next stage occurs when glycogen is completed depleted. Gluconeogenesis completely takes over and ketones begin to be produced in low quantities. This is called the gluconeogenic phase.

As the body does not get supplied with sufficient carbohydrates, ketosis occurs. This is characterized by a decrease in the use of non-carbohydrate components like amino acids to create energy and a complete shift to prioritizing the production of ketones.

Ketones are formed in the liver as fat cells get broken down in a process called ketogenesis. The first ketone that is produced is acetoacetate. Acetoacetate is then converted to beta-hydroxybutyrate, or BHB for short, and acetone. As your body adapts to gaining energy from ketosis, BHB becomes the most common ketone. When you full adapted to ketosis, ketones provide up to 50% of the body's base energy while catering to up to 70% of the brain's energy needs.

How Ketosis Causes Weight Loss

It might be difficult to understand how a diet can recommend the consumption of fat to lose weight while traditional diets preach the exact opposite. This might seem like madness to an outside observer. However, taking a closer look shows that the ketogenic diet promotes the burning of fat to form ketones, which leads to natural weight loss.

Also, because of the foods that are recommended for consumption are high in healthy fat and protein, the practitioner is left feeling fuller and more satisfied after every meal. This leads to not overeating and therefore, better weight reduction and metabolic health.

It also creates a reduction in appetite as well so that the person does not overeat by indiscriminately reaching for snacks during the day. Unfortunately, the most convenient snacks that are available happen to be those loaded in carbohydrates. Even if the person has healthy snack options but indulges is sweets too often, the results are often linked to weight gain. On the ketogenic diet, appetite is curbed to lessen the likelihood of reaching for unhealthy snacks or for snacking too much.

One of the most common problem areas that people experience when losing weight is the belly area. Belly fat consists of visceral fat, which is a type of fat that encases internal organs around the abdominal area. The build-up of this type of fat has been linked to the development of type 2 diabetes and heart disease. The ketogenic diet makes it possible to eliminate visceral fat because visceral fat production has been closely linked to the consumption of carbohydrates and refined sugars. Both of these are discouraged on the ketogenic diet which leads to a reduction of the development of this type of fat and therefore, weight loss in the abdominal area as well as all over the body.

Other Benefits of Ketosis

Ketosis is not just about fat burning. It has many serious and positive implications for your health and wellness. They include:

• The stimulation of mitochondrial production. Mitochondria are the part of body cells that generate the chemical energy needed to facilitate the cell's biochemical reactions. New mitochondria are synthesized in cells that used ketones as a fuel. This is especially prominent in brain cells. The formation of more mitochondria helps improve energy production and the overall health of cells.

• Ketones function similarly to an antioxidant. An antioxidant is a substance that removes potentially damaging oxidizing agents from forming in the body. Oxidation is a chemical process that occurs in cells and can produce free radicals, which are chemicals that damage cells. Vitamin C and E are popular antioxidants. Ketones produce less reactive oxygen and therefore, less free radicals than sugar and thus protects cells from damage.

• The protection and regeneration of nervous system cells. Ketosis aids in regenerating damaged nerve cells as well as preserving the function of aging nerve cells.

• Aids in preventing certain cancers. Most cancer cells cannot use ketones as fuel and therefore, die because they have nothing to facilitate their growth. This aids the immune system in removing them from the body.

• Aids in improving brain function. There have been promising studies on how the ketogenic diet and ketosis improve the brain function in people with autism, epilepsy, Alzheimer's disease, and Parkinson's disease, This can be attributed to the fact that the brain uses energy derived from ketones more effectively than it does with energy obtained from sugar. Ketosis also has an inhibitory effect on nerve cells, which makes the brain less excitable and therefore, more efficient in its function.

• Triggers the process of autophagy. Autophagy means "self-eating". It is the process whereby the body cleans out damaged cells and toxins in addition to regenerating new, healthier cells. Damaged cells and toxins accumulate over time if this process does not work efficiently. This causes several negative effects such as inducing dementia, increasing the risk of developing certain cancers and accelerating aging. Consuming more fat on the ketogenic diet activates autophagy because your cells become more efficient at cleaning out old cells and regenerating new ones once it stops relying on carbohydrates to provide energy.

Exercising on the Keto Vegan Diet

Exercise and dieting go hand-in-hand if a person wants to live a healthy lifestyle and to lose weight in a safe and sustainable way. Experiencing the keto flu at the initial stages of starting this diet may make it difficult to partake in a normal exercise routine but long-term, practicing the keto vegan diet can actually improve your athletic performance, especially in endurance sports.

In the first few weeks of practicing the ketogenic vegan diet, it is recommended that you start with light exercises as your body begins to adjust to this fat-adapted way of eating. Such exercises include light hiking, walking, cycling, and yoga. It is also recommended that you stick to relatively flat surfaces as dizziness is a common symptom of the keto flu. No matter what exercise you choose to partake in or what stage in your ketogenic diet you are in be sure to be aware of your water intake so that you do not become dehydrated. You should also increase your mineral and electrolyte consumption accordingly to your level of exercise.

Chapter 3: The benefits

We know that there are several benefits associated with the keto diet and similar is for a vegan keto diet. By making vegan keto a part of your life, you will help yourself against illness. It might help to prevent several diseases.

High Blood Pressure

If you are facing high blood pressure, then eating vegan keto would be useful for you. In some cases, this diet may give you a little relief from the problem whereas in some cases it would completely treat it. Even if you are taking medications to handle high blood pressure then start eating a vegan keto diet. The relief given by vegan keto diet may take from days to months. When you start with the diet symptoms of improvement, appear and then the disease is adequately treated. The patients who start eating vegan keto diet are recommended to take "Salt and Bouillon" along vegan keto diet. This provides you extra fluids and salts so that you may not face early side effects of low carb diet like a headache. But if you are suffering a high blood pressure despite medication then do not take extra salts and fluids. It may be harmful as it would raise blood pressure further.

Fights Obesity

We know that the ketogenic diet plan has come up with the primary aim to reduce a person's weight. Every meal plan that is designed by dieticians has a purpose. Over here ketogenic diet was designed for getting rid of extra pounds that you have gained. Similarly, vegan keto offers us the benefit. Though it is difficult to adjust your carbs while eating vegan keto diet but it can be done by putting in greater intellect. Ketogenic diet plan helps us to fight obesity in a way that it burns all the extra fats gained on your body. How does it happen? As we know that a ketogenic diet plan is a modernly designed diet that is high in fats, moderate with proteins, and low at carbs. When our body is in a normal state, it utilizes carbohydrates as a source of energy. We can also say that sugars are the immediate source of energy in our body because they are quickly metabolized. But when we start eating keto or vegan keto diet, we provide fewer carbs to our collection. When there are no carbs in the body that could be used for energy, then large reservoirs are used. Fats are metabolized, ketone bodies are formed in the liver and are transported to body organs for use. In keto, we eat fats that are basically from an animal source. But in the case of vegan keto, we do not eat an animal-based diet, so all of the fats are taken up by plant-based foods. When the extra fat on your body is burnt you lose weight. This process continues if you follow the meal plan strictly.

Improved skin Usually you might face skin problems. Skin problems are mostly due to hormonal imbalances occurring in your body. When you begin with a vegan keto diet, you would see a surprising improvement in your skin condition. This is because during vegan keto you only take a plant-based diet. Many of the fruits and vegetables are rich in antioxidants which would help you to have brighter and healthier skin.

High Levels of Adiponectin Helps Type 2 Diabetes

Lipids stored on your body are mostly as adipose tissues. These storage tissues are not inert but secrete different kinds of bioactive molecules. They are called adipokines. Adiponectin is among those adipokines which have an inverse relation with insulin resistance. High serum levels of adiponectin helped insulin resistance in type 2 diabetic patients. Adiponectin is inversely related to abdominal obesity as well. Whenever you start with a keto diet plan or vegan keto diet plan, it gives you several health benefits. Type 2 diabetes is the ailment in which insulin resistance is developed in the body. Disturbed insulin levels negatively impact blood sugar regulation of your body. Vegan keto is effective for insulin resistant diabetic patients.

Improves Inflammation

It can be said that a vegan keto diet is the best to reduce inflammation. In vegan keto diet we reduce the number of carbs taken by the body. The vegan keto diet helps us to get rid of extra fluids. Along with this, it helps to increase the level of ketone bodies in your body. Beta-Hydroxybutyrate is among those ketones which help to lower the inflammation in your body. This ketone helps to deactivate those chemicals that are responsible for inflammation. Your body could continue the process of healing without feeling pain.

Improves Heart Health

A vegan keto diet is adequate for your heart health. It would help your heart to beat healthily. We know that in vegan keto diet we do not consume animal products. The food we eat is only plant-based. It helps us to mitigate cholesterol. A high cholesterol level of your body is the primary driver to cardiovascular diseases. It could even lead to myocardial infarction. To keep your heart healthy and to let your blood run rapidly within your vessels, eat a vegan keto diet. Saturated fats are not suitable for your health. When you are eating vegan keto, you do not consume saturated fats. This is effective to fight against high cholesterol levels of your body. When eating vegan keto, you do not face high dietary cholesterol and low-density-lipid cholesterol. This would eventually lead to improved heart health.

Here one thing to be noticed is that vegan could not only leas to improved heart health. This is because some foods are vegan keto-friendly but would raise the cholesterol level. They might increase the level of salts and fats in your body. So everybody who wants to try a new diet plan must consult the doctor before opting for something new. When we think to begin with vegan foods that are plant derived. The quick answer that comes from our mind is that this diet would be undoubtedly effective for weight loss. But the goodness of vegan keto is not only confined to weight loss. It gives you several other benefits if your company it with other nutrient-pack alternatives.

Chapter 4: What to eat on keto vegan diet

If we think vegan and keto as two independent approaches, they would seem opposite, as they are. Vegan and Keto eaters do not have much in common. One plan demands to eat a lot of meat while in the other case we have to refrain from meat entirely. In one case we have to load up on carbs, while another example we think of plans to stay away from carbs. We can say that that vegan and keto diet independently are like North and South poles. Two opposite ends that never meet! But what if we try to combine these two ideas? It is difficult, but it's not impossible. All you have to do is to walk in the fine line rather than a promenade.

Vegans do not eat food that is animal based. During the vegan diet, you have to avoid all kinds of poultry foods as well. We might eat a vegan diet for a health reason or due to some ethical reasons. Keto diet was brought to is in 1920 to treat epilepsy. But then it became a modern trend, and here we sum up vegan and keto. The answer is somehow like low carbs, moderate proteins, high fats, and no animal-based feed.

During the vegan keto diet the person has to stay within the following requirements:

• Minimum carbohydrates

• A lot of fats that are obtained from plants

• Sufficient plant-based proteins

Fruits

Fruits are not only delicious but are a good source of vitamins and minerals. They are full of nutrients. When eating grains, you can get a lot of water that fulfill the water deficiencies of your body and helps keep your body hydrated. Watermelons are mostly water that is 92%. A lot of water helps your kidneys to work efficiently. People who eat fruits frequently are less likely to develop chronic diseases. Tomatoes are used in salads and different food items. They are rich in antioxidants. Citrus fruits contain a high content of Vitamin C. It plays a role in the strengthening of teeth and gums. It is also suitable for blood cells. Olives are obtained from olive trees. They are eaten in pesto, salads, and tapenade. Coconuts are high in MCTs whereas Avocados have an unbelievable abundance of fats.

Fridge Staples which are Vegan Keto Friendly

We must know what to put in the fridge so that it could be most beneficial for us. Apple cider vinegar is made by using fermented apple juice. It is used in dressings and salads. Apples are crushed to draw out the liquid out of them after which bacteria are added to them. Dairy-Free yogurt is a special preparation that is for lactose-intolerant people. It is made for two purposes one is for the betterment of those who can't metabolize lactic acid, and the other reason is those on a vegan keto diet. Similar is for dairy-free cheeses. They are for those who can't tolerate lactose. All the cheeses that are prepared from alternate sources than the original do not possess similar taste. Pickles are also made by fermentation and are consumed along with meals for a better experience. As they contain vegetables mostly so can be said as vegan keto friendly. Tofu is commonly known as bean curd which is vegan keto friendly.

Pantry Staples which are Vegan Keto Friendly

Staple foods are those food items that are eaten regularly. They include different flours, powders, kinds of milk, and extracts. Over here we have a list of those ingredients that are frequently used in preparing our daily meals. When we are on a vegan keto diet, we have to stay low at carbs. The flour that is obtained from wheat is high in starch. Starch is a rich source of carbohydrates so to replace wheat flour we have different alternatives like almond flour, coconut flour, and psyllium husk. As we can't take dairy products, we need a replacement for milk. The duty is performed by coconut milk. Apart from milk and flour are other staples that are used regularly. All of the above items in the list are vegan keto friendly.

Vegan Keto Meal Staples

In vegan keto diet we are eating foods that are high in fats, low in carbs, and moderate at proteins. And they are derived from a plant source. The meal can be defined as a preparation that is a combination of different ingredients to satisfy your hunger.

Snacks are what we daily eat. Vegan Keto diet gives us food items that are friendly to the diet plan and are enough to meet our craving at once. We have two types of noodles, herbs and spices, flakes, and seaweed. All of these ingredients can be taken alone or can be used in the preparation of various recipes which are made by using vegan keto friendly food items. Shirataki noodles are with zero calories. They are mostly water and a little fiber. Traces of proteins are present in these noodles. Kelp is a source of Vitamin A, Vitamin B, and Vitamin E. Kelp contains the highest concentration of calcium among the naturally occurring foods. Here we have kelp noodles and kelp flakes which are full of nutrition. Then comes the seaweed which belongs to algae. They are edible and are enriched with fiber. The plant also contains a high amount of iron and calcium. Edamame is referred to as immature beans. They are added to different food preparations. They could also be eaten after boiling in water and sprinkling with salt.

Foods to Avoid on Vegan Keto Diet

The combined version of two diet plans; ketogenic diet plan and vegan diet plan has some restrictions. We have to follow those restrictions to stay in the premises of vegan keto diet plan. During this plan, we can't eat anything that is obtained from an animal source. We have to eat a lot of fats from a plant source, a limited amount of carbs and a moderate quantity of proteins. During the diet plan we have to avoid:

Meat , Eggs , Poultry , Dairy , Fish

Meat has been the food of humans for decades. It is the flesh of animals that we eat to satisfy our hunger. Some people do not eat meat because of ethical or religious reasons, and some might do not like meat. But the rest of the world is crazy over it. Most commonly people all over the world eat the meat of chicken, sheep, pig, rabbit, and cattle. Meat has water, fats, and proteins in it. The eggs we eat are mostly of hens. However, duck and quail eggs are also eaten. They are a rich source of proteins but aren't allowed when you are following a vegan keto diet plan. Poultry gives us different types of meat that we ought not to eat as well. Dairy products are made using the milk of mammals. Fish is seafood, and as we can't eat anything animal-based, we have to refrain from dairy products and all types of fishes as well.

Gelatin

Gelatin is derived from the body parts of animals. It is a colorless, tasteless translucent material. Gelatin is hydrolyzed collagen. The gelatin exhibits two types of appearances in two different conditions. When it is dry, it looks brittle whereas when moist it gives a cohesive look and texture. Gelatinous substances work similarly as gelatin. When the protein fibrils of collagen are irreversibly hydrolyzed, it gives us gelatin. The molecular weight of these protein fibrils fluctuates within a broad range and depends on the method we use for protein denaturation. Gelatin has a lot of uses, but it is widely used as a gelling agent in foods, medicines, vitamins, and capsules. It is also used in cosmetics.

Some dessert preparations also contain gelatin like marshmallows, gummy candies, yogurts if various kinds, and ice-cream dips. Dry weight if gelatin claims it to be 98-99% protein. A little number of other nutrients might be present in gelatin which depends on the raw materials used for its preparation and processing technique employed.

Refined Sugar

Sugar is nothing but carbohydrate that our body may utilize to produce glucose but the way through which we obtain it matters. We prepare refined sugar by using sugarcane or sugar beet. We extract the sugar out of them by following extraction methods. Natural sugar is fructose whereas refined sugar is a combination of fructose and sucrose. We use this sugar as white sugar or brown sugar. It has various uses in our cooking recipes to sweeten everything. Food manufacturers add the chemically produced sugar to foods which is not the part of our vegan keto diet plan. High-fructose corn syrup, cane sugar, caramel, maltose, dextrose, invert sugar, and corn syrup are some examples of refined sugar. When we eat these refined sugars, our carbohydrate level might exceed up to devastating levels, and we won't be able to stay low at carbs. The motive of our vegan keto diet plan would be tremored. Eating refined sugar will eventually lead to weight gain because the fat will accumulate on your body. Excess of fats may cause cardiovascular problems. High sugars are also responsible for androgen secretion and inflammation which might lead to acne. As we would become obese, insulin resistance would be developed, and hence diabetes would result. All of these factors can support cancer. We might also face depression and along with this a faster aging process. Moreover, we would start losing our stamina, and all of our energy would be drained rapidly.

Grains

During vegan, keto diet avoids eating legumes, beans, pasta, and wheat. All wheat products are also avoided. Though all of these products are plant-derived, we will refrain from eating them. This is because of the high carbohydrate content of these. Wheat has 71% carbohydrate content, 13% water, 13% proteins which are mostly gluten and 1.5% fats. It also provides us some vitamins and minerals. All the food products that contain wheat must not be eaten during you are following a vegan keto diet plan. They include porridge, biscuits, crackers, pancakes, pasta, bread, cakes, cookies, donuts, muffins, rolls, pizza, and many other yummy food items. As all of these would shatter our specified limits of carb intake. Do not eat during you are following a vegan keto diet plan. Legumes should be avoided in vegan keto diet plan because of the anti-nutrients they contain. As they are high in carbs, it would disturb our normal plan.

Starchy Vegetables

Though vegetables are good for us as they provide us a lot of vitamins and minerals during vegan keto diet, we have to avoid starchy vegetables. They include corn, yams, beans, and potatoes. Starch is a quite complex carbohydrate molecule. This is because of several sugar molecules are joined in it. Starchy and non-starchy vegetables both are full of nutrients, but we can't eat starchy vegetables while being on ketosis. During ketosis, our body uses fats as a source of energy rather than carbs. This is because we limit the carb supply. Eating starchy vegetables would disturb the process.

High-Carb Nuts

Nuts are nutritious and delicious. We can eat them raw or can add them to different food preparations. They are expensive to buy so buy them in bulk and store properly so that they may not go rancid. But during vegan keto, we must not eat foods high in carbs. Avoid eating pistachios, cashews, and chestnuts. These three nuts have a greater carb content. Chestnuts have 29.7g, cashews have 16.8g, and pistachios have 6.8g carbs in each 100g of serving. Peanuts are also rich in carbs so do not make it a part of your food when you are on a vegan keto diet plan.

Partially Hydrogenated Oils & Refined Vegetable Oils

Oil is hydrogenated to increase its shelf life. During the process, we convert unsaturated fats to solid fat by the addition of hydrogen gas. This process is also used to save money. During the process of partial hydrogenation, we obtain trans fats. This raises the level of bad cholesterol in our body and lowers the level of good cholesterol. Trans fats are responsible for this which are readily made during partial hydrogenation whereas we do not face such problem during complete hydrogenation. Refined vegetable oils are prepared by using plant seeds. They are highly dangerous to us. This oil contains polyunsaturated fatty acids. At room temperature this oil remains liquid but when it is exposed to light disaster occurs. Free radicals are formed that can be the reason for causing cancer. Oxidation occurs when they are exposed to light which leads to the formation of free radicals. So we must avoid using refined vegetable oils in every case.

Chapter 5: Breakfast

Avocado with halloumi cheese

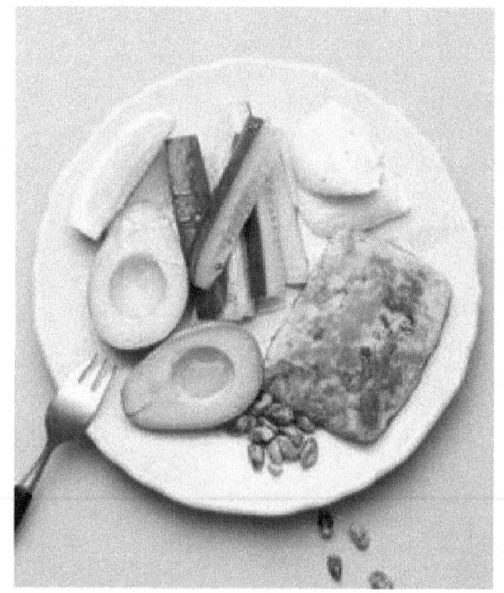

Preparation time: 10 minutes

Cooking time: 4 minutes

Servings: 12

Ingredients:

1 avocado

140 g halloumi cheese

1 teaspoon butter for frying

1 tablespoon of olive oil

1/4 cup sour cream

¼ fresh cucumber

1 tbsp pistachio nuts

salt and pepper

¼ lemon (optional)

Direction

Halloumi cheese cut into slices, heat butter in a frying pan and fry the cheese until golden brown.

While the cheese is frying, cut the avocado and remove the stone.

Cut the cucumbers into sticks and place with avocado on a plate - sprinkle with lemon juice, olive oil and sprinkle with salt and pepper.

Serve with fried cheese and sour cream.

If you don't like cucumber, you can easily replace it with another crunchy vegetable, e.g. celery, radish, kohlrabi.

Vegetarian pizza recipe

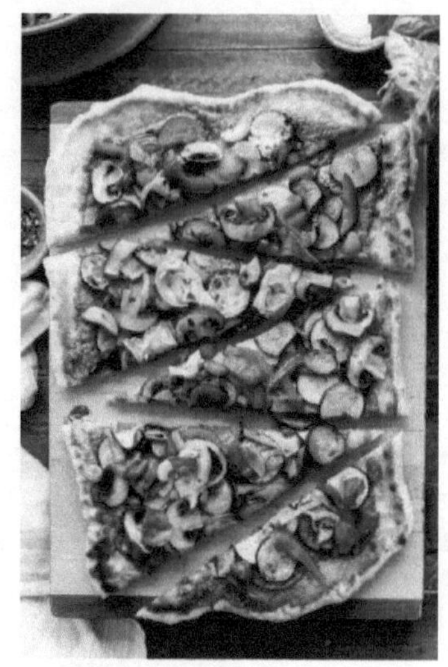

Preparation time: 10 minutes

Cooking time: 10 minutes

Servings: 12

Cake Products:

2 eggs

½ cup mayonnaise

¾ cup of almond flour

1 tablespoon of plantain husk

1 teaspoon of baking powder

½ tsp salt

Products-Extras:

50-60 g mushrooms

1 tablespoon of green pesto

2 tablespoons of olive oil

½ cup 18% cream

¾ cup grated cheese

salt and pepper

arugula

Direction

Preheat to 175 ° C in the oven.

Combine well the eggs and mayonnaise, add to the dough the remaining ingredients, combine and wait for 5 minutes.

Then add on your hands a few drops of oil and evenly spread the dough on a baking tray lined with baking paper. The thickness should be no more than 1 cm.

Bake until the dough starts to brown lightly for 10 minutes. Clear from the oven and let it cool down. Cut the mushrooms in thin slices at this moment.

Put the cream on the cooled cake and add oil and spices to the pesto.

Sprinkle with the aged cheese and finish with the mushrooms. Place the pizza 5-10 minutes in the oven until the cheese is dissolved. Serve with salad from the rocket.

Spinach lasagne with zucchini

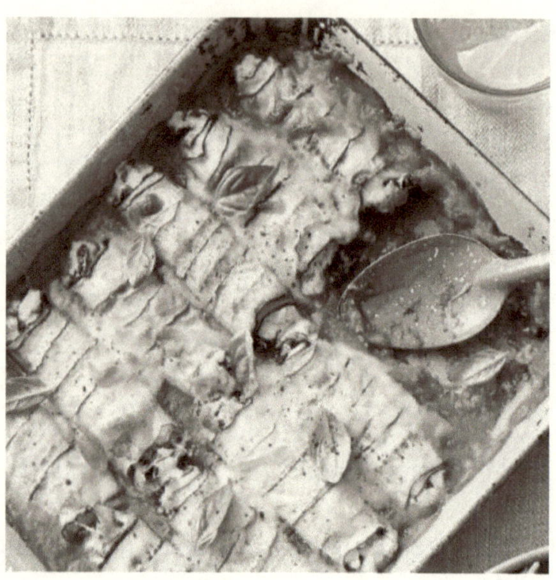

Preparation time: 10 minutes

Cooking time: 4 minutes

(9 servings)

Ingredients :

4 medium courgettes

450 g mozzarella - crumbled

1 teaspoon parsley - chopped

1 tablespoon of olive oil

½ onions - finely chopped

4 garlic cloves - crushed

420 g ricotta

1 large egg

½ cup grated Parmesan cheese

2 tablespoons of tomato paste

1 can of tomatoes without skin

Salt and black pepper to taste

1 tablespoon of fresh chopped basil

3 cups fresh spinach

Direction

In a saucepan in olive oil, fry the onion, add garlic and fry - make sure that the garlic does not burn. Then add the tomato concentrate and chopped canned tomatoes mix well. Season with salt and pepper. Cook for 25-30 minutes on medium heat so that the sauce evaporates slightly. Finally, remove from heat and add fresh basil and spinach. Mix well.

Heat the oven to 190 ° C. Cut zucchini into thin slices, slicing lengthwise - a potato peeler or sharp knife is great for this. Arrange the slices of zucchini in one layer on a baking tray lined with baking paper. Bake for 5-8 minutes. Remove from the oven, wait 5 minutes and drain the excess water with a paper towel. This part is very important so that lasagna is not watery.

In a medium bowl, mix the ricotta cheese, parmesan cheese and egg well. Line the bottom of a 22x30cm ovenproof dish or baking dish with ⅓ tomato sauce and spinach, ⅓ zucchini slices, then ⅓ cheese mix and ⅓ grated mozzarella cheese.

Perform the next 2 layers in the same way. There must be mozzarella on top. Cover the heat-resistant dish with aluminum foil and bake for 30 minutes. Then remove the foil and bake for another 10-15 minutes.

Let stand for about 10 minutes before serving. Garnish with parsley.

Keto rice with cheddar cheese

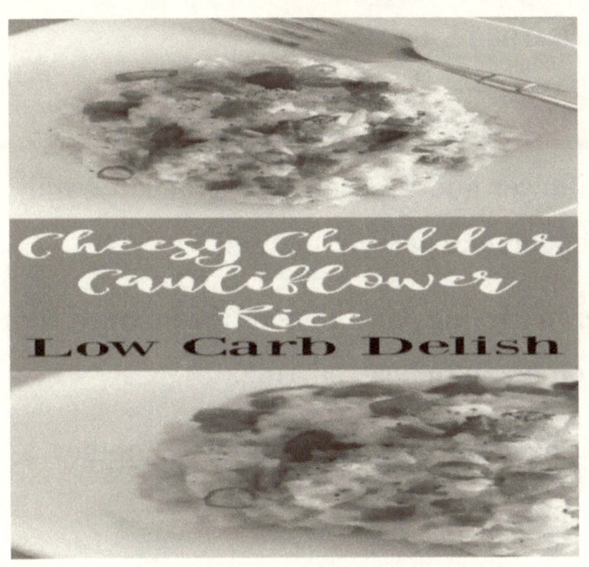

Preparation time: 10 minutes

Cooking time: 30 minutes

(1 portion)

Ingredient :

3 cups of grated cauliflower

1 cup grated broccoli

1 tablespoon of butter

1/2 teaspoon salt

1/4 teaspoon pepper

1/4 teaspoon garlic powder

a pinch of ground nutmeg

1/2 cup shredded spicy cheddar cheese

1/4 cup mascarpone

Direction

Grate cauliflower and broccoli on a grater put into a bowl and add salt, pepper, and garlic - mix well.

Heat butter in a frying pan and pour the mixture, fry for about 6-8 minutes on medium heat, stirring.

Then add cheddar cheese and fry for another 2-3 minutes, stirring.

Combine it with mascarpone cheese to achieve a creamy consistency. Season according to your taste.

Serve hot.

Caprese

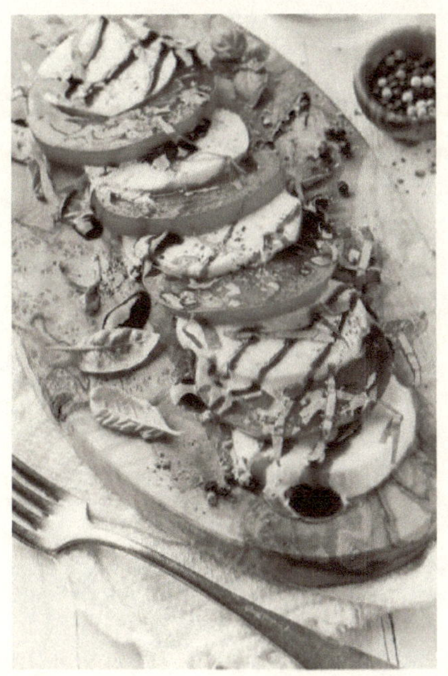

Preparation time: 10 minutes

Cooking time: 40 minutes

(1 serving)

Ingredients:

60 g cherry tomatoes

60 g mini mozzarella

1 teaspoon of green pesto

salt and pepper

Direction

Cut in half the tomatoes and balls of mozzarella. Add and whisk the pesto.

To taste the salt and the pepper. New basil or chopped parsley can be added.

Wege pasta

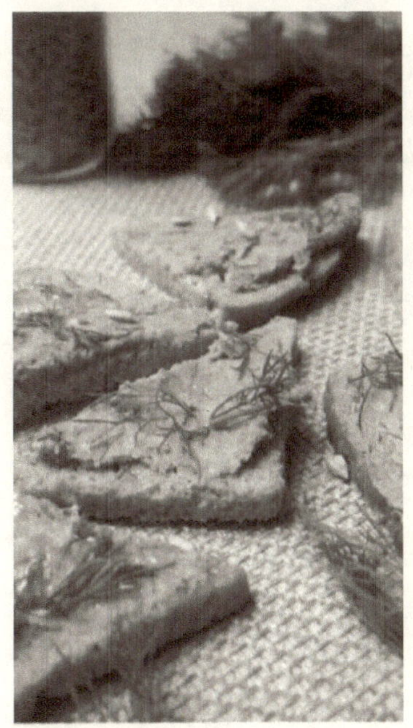

Preparation time: 10 minutes

Cooking time: 40 minutes

Servings: 12

 (2 servings)

Ingredient :

4 eggs

150 g Philadelphia cream cheese

½ tsp salt

40 ml (20 g) of ground ovoid husk

Sauce

100 g Blue Blue cheese

100 g Philadelphia cream cheese

30 g butter

1 pinch of pepper

For serving

2 tablespoons of roasted nuts

60 ml freshly grated Parmesan cheese

Direction

Preheat the oven to 150 ° C.

Mix the eggs, cheese, and salt into a liquid dough. Continue mixing by adding plantain husk. Let the dough rest for 2 minutes.

Place the dough on a parchment paper-lined baking sheet. Use a rolling pin to put another parchment on top and flatten it.

Place the parchment cake in the oven and bake for 10-12 minutes. Heat the paper and cut it.

Cut the pasta with a pizza cutter or a sharp knife into thin strips. Place in the refrigerator.

Until serving, refresh the pasta: heat the pasta in a microwave or oven sauce for 30 seconds. Melt the blue cheese gently over low heat in a small saucepan, stirring periodically.

Apply cream cheese and, for a few minutes, blend well.

Remove butter and mix it together. Don't put to a boil the sauce.

Use the noodles to eat. Top with freshly grated Parmesan cheese and roasted nuts.

Microwave Quick Keto Bread

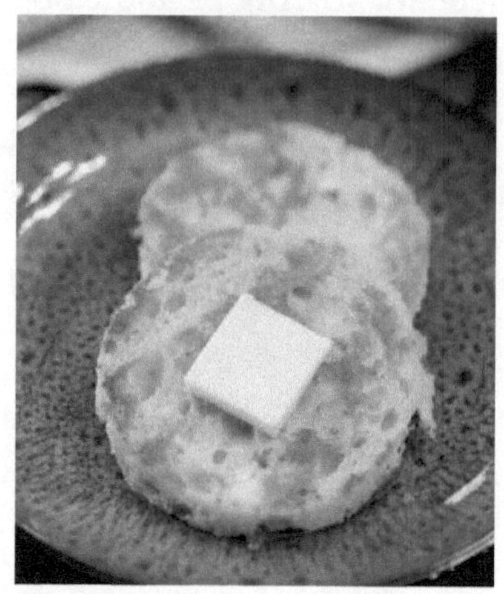

Preparation time: 10 minutes

Cooking time: 4 minutes

Servings: 12

Ingredients:

3 tbsp almond flour

½ tsp psyllium powder

½ tsp baking powder

A pinch of salt

1 tbsp ghee

1 large egg

Direction

Add the dry ingredients to a small bowl, then butter and egg. Mix well.

Lubricate the microwave, mug, or small bowl, and add the batter.

Put the bread in the microwave for 80-100 seconds.

Gently place the bread on a cutting board and cut in half.

Pork cutlets

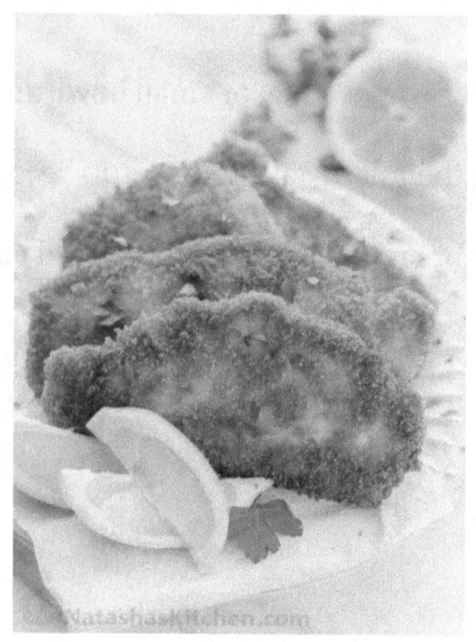

Ingredients:

450 g minced pork

1 tsp ground sage

1 tsp dried rosemary

1 tsp salt

1 tsp ground pepper

¼ tsp ground fennel

⅛ tsp chili powder

1 tbsp olive oil for frying

Direction

Mix in a bowl all the ingredients except the oil.

Divide the mixture into 6 balls and form cutlets.

Pour oil into a large frying pan with a nonstick coating over high heat and fry the patties for 2-3 minutes on each side until cooked.

Shakshuka with goat cheese

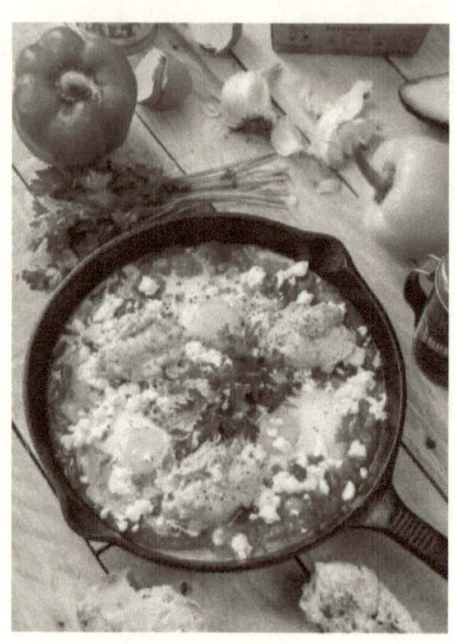

Preparation time: 10 minutes

Cooking time: 30 minutes

Servings: 12

Ingredients

¼ cup olive oil

3 cups chopped greens

1 medium yellow onion, diced

1 medium jalapeno chopped

½ medium green bell pepper, diced

4 garlic cloves, minced

1 tbsp paprika

½ tsp chopped red pepper

Salt and pepper to taste

800 g sugar-free tomato puree

6 large eggs

113 g goat cheese

Direction

Preheat the oven to 204 degrees. Heat the pan over medium heat and heat the olive oil.

Once it is hot, add herbs, onions, jalapenos, green bell peppers, and garlic. Cook everything until soft, then add paprika, chopped red pepper, salt, and black pepper.

Add the tomato puree and continue cooking until the sauce is pleasant and hot. Turn off the fire.

Using a spoon, make holes in the sauce, then break into each egg.

Put the pan in the oven and bake for 5 minutes.

Top crumble the goat cheese.

Low Carb Chocolate Muffins

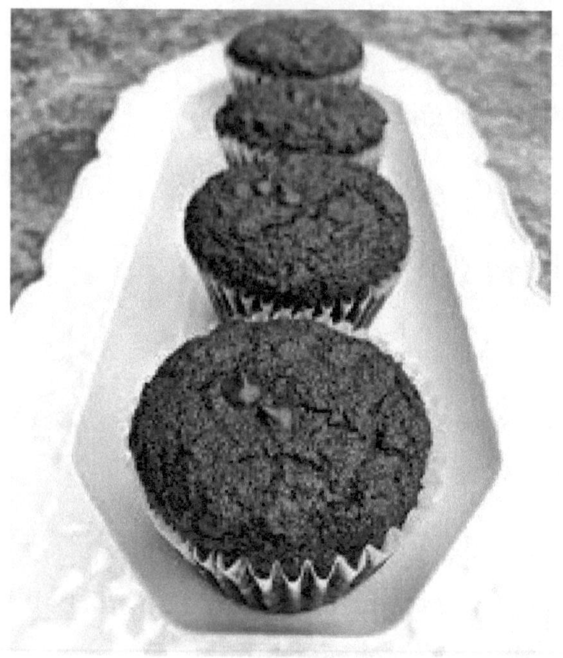

Preparation time: 10 minutes

Cooking time: 45 minutes

Servings: 12

Ingredients:

226.8 g almond flour

0.03 kg coconut flour

2 tsp baking powder

A pinch of salt

113.4 g unsalted butter (melted)

⅓ cup stevia

1 tsp vanilla essence

2 large eggs

⅓ cups of chocolate drops without sugar (minimum 80% cocoa). Or you can just grind low-carb chocolate.

Direction

Preheat the oven to 180 degrees. Layout the baking sheet with parchment paper.

Combine almond and coconut flour, baking powder and salt.

Beat with a mixer the oil, sweetener, and vanilla essence for 5-8 minutes, until light and fluffy. Add one egg at a time and then flour. Mix well.

Add chocolate and whisk again.

Put the dough on a piece of parchment paper and squeeze it into a circle about 2.5 cm thick.

Cut like a pizza into 8 slices. Gently peel the slices with a spatula or knife.

Bake for 15-20 minutes until the buns begin to brown. When pressed to the center, they should be a little soft.

Leave on a baking sheet for 10 minutes.

Creamy Cucumber Sandwiches

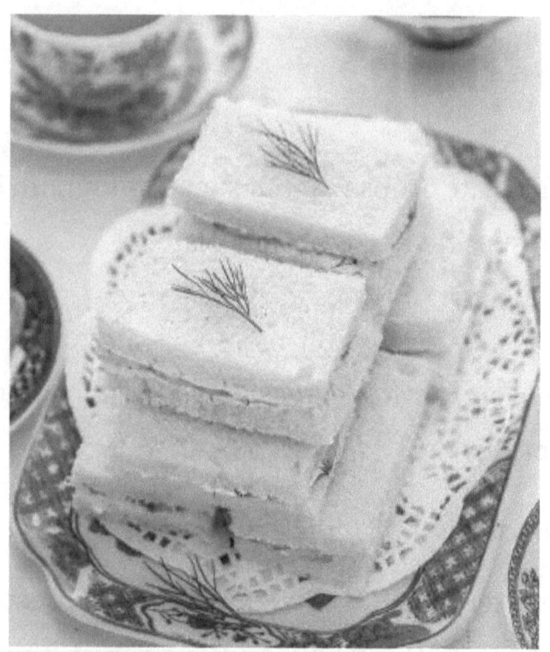

Ingredients:

85 g cream cheese

1 medium cucumber

1 tbsp sour cream

1/8 tsp salt

1 pinch of pepper

1/8 tsp garlic powder

Almond flour bread or other low-carb bread

Direction

Grate the cucumber and let the excess liquid drain.

Mix cream cheese, cucumber, and sour cream until smooth. Season with salt, pepper and garlic powder.

Cut the slices of low-carb bread in half to make them thinner. Put the cucumber mixture on the bottom slice and cover it with the top slice. Cut in half.

Coconut flour biscuits with cheese

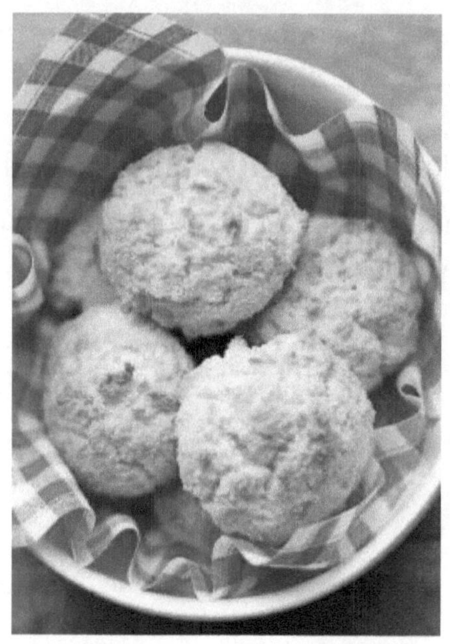

Preparation time: 10 minutes

Cooking time: 4 minutes

Servings: 12

Ingredients

4 eggs

56.75 g melted butter

0.25 tsp salt

2 tsp garlic powder

0.25 tsp onion powder

40 g coconut flour

0.5 tsp xanthan gum (optional)

0.25 tsp baking powder

56.5 g chopped cheddar cheese

Cooking

Beat eggs, oil, salt, garlic, and onion powder together.

In a separate bowl, mix coconut flour with baking powder and xanthan gum.

Add the dry ingredients to the egg mixture. Beat and add cheese.

Place the dough with a tablespoon on a greased baking sheet.

Bake at 204 degrees for 15 minutes.

Breakfast in a cup with ham and cheese

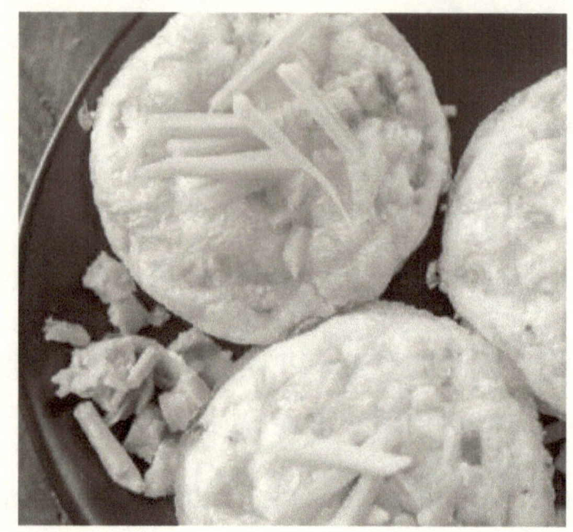

Preparation time: 10 minutes

Cooking time: 30 minutes

Servings: 12

Ingredients:

12 slices of ham

4 eggs

1 tbsp grated parmesan cheese

1 tbsp chopped parsley

1 tsp olive oil for lubrication

1/4 tsp sea salt

1/4 tsp black pepper

Direction

Preheat the oven to 176 degrees.

Divide 12 slices of ham between 4 muffin or ramekin molds (greased with olive oil).

Break each egg into each pan, season with salt and pepper, and bake for 20 minutes.

Serve immediately, sprinkled with parmesan and chopped parsley

Coconut flour biscuits with cheese

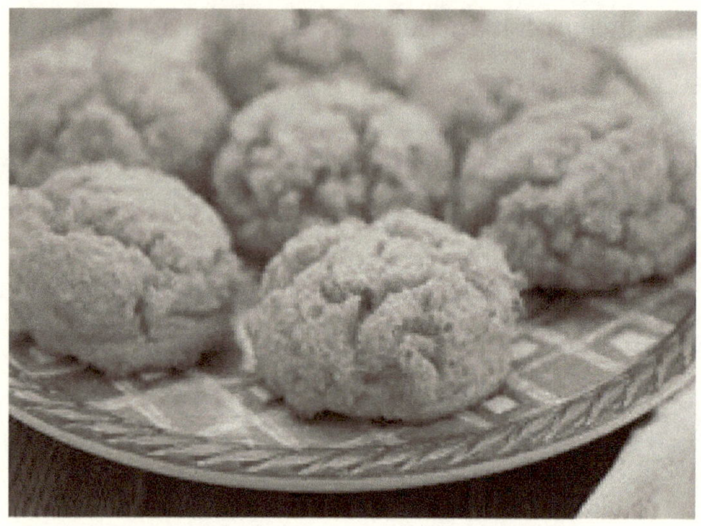

Preparation time: 10 minutes

Cooking time: 4 minutes

Servings: 12

Ingredients:

4 eggs

56.75 g melted butter

0.25 tsp salt

2 tsp garlic powder

0.25 tsp onion powder

40 g coconut flour

0.5 tsp xanthan gum (optional)

0.25 tsp baking powder

56.5 g chopped cheddar cheese

Direction

Beat eggs, oil, salt, garlic, and onion powder together.

In a separate bowl, mix coconut flour with baking powder and xanthan gum.

Add the dry ingredients to the egg mixture. Beat and add cheese.

Place the dough with a tablespoon on a greased baking sheet.

Bake at 204 degrees for 15 minutes.

Aerial keto waffles

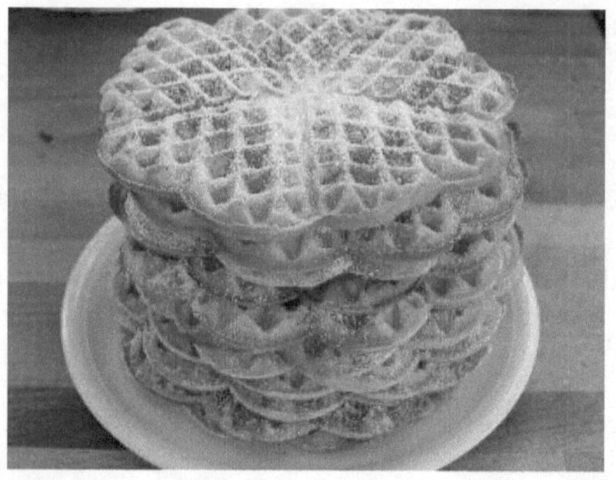

Preparation time: 10 minutes

Cooking time: 40 minutes

Servings: 12

Ingredients:

1 1/2 cup almond flour

2 tbsp coconut flour

1/2 tsp baking powder

1 tsp baking soda

2 large whole eggs

1 tbsp maple extract

2 tbsp stevia or another low-carb sweetener

2 tbsp melted butter

1 1/4 cup unsweetened milk to your taste

Direction

Put all the ingredients in a large bowl. Mix well with a spatula or mixer until smooth. Leave on for 5 minutes.

Preheat the waffle iron and grease with a nonstick spray, butter or coconut oil.

Pour the dough into waffle iron and cook for 3-4 minutes until golden on each side. Place the finished waffles in the oven so that they are crispy while you cook the remaining waffles.

For the topping, try homemade almond butter, cream cheese, and strawberries, or whipped coconut cream.

Keto omelet with minced meat

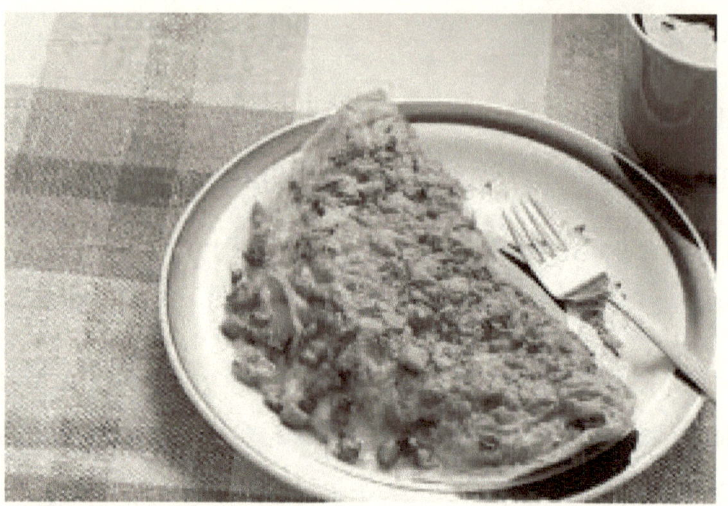

Preparation time: 10 minutes

Cooking time: 4 minutes

Servings: 12

Ingredients:

85.05 g pork or ground beef

2 eggs

1 tbsp fat cream

1 tsp hot low carb sauce

2 tbsp cheddar cheese

2 tsp olive oil (individually)

Sea salt and pepper to taste

1 tsp chopped green onions

Direction

Break the eggs into a blender. Pour in heavy cream, and season with salt and pepper. Mix everything together until smooth.

Heat 1 teaspoon of olive oil in a pan, add the minced meat and cook for 5 minutes or until brown.

Add hot sauce, season with salt and pepper, and cook another 1-2 minutes. Set aside.

Place the pan over medium heat and pour the remaining olive oil. When the oil is warm, carefully pour the beaten eggs into the pan, cover and leave until cooked.

After the omelet is fried, put the minced meat on one side, sprinkle with chopped cheese, and then roll the omelet.

Cover and cook over low heat for another 1-2 minutes until the cheese melts.

Transfer to a dish and sprinkle with chopped green onions.

Peanut Butter Pancakes

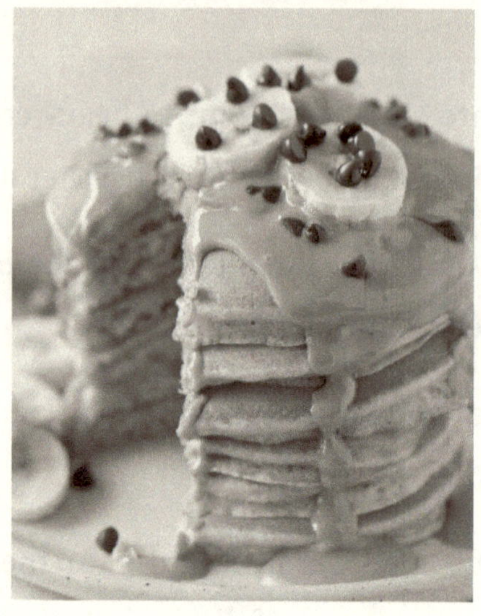

Preparation time: 10 minutes

Cooking time: 40 minutes

Servings: 12

Ingredients:

1 1/4 cup peanut flour

2 tsp stevia or erythritis

1 tbsp baking powder

1/2 tsp salt

1 1/2 cup unsweetened almond or coconut milk

2 eggs

1/4 cup natural peanut butter

1 tsp vanilla extract

Direction

In a medium bowl, mix dry ingredients. In a separate bowl, mix the wet ingredients until smooth.

Add wet ingredients to dry ingredients and beat until batter forms. If the dough is too thick, add milk.

Put 1 tablespoon in a heated pan, and brown until brown on both sides.

Tuna Egg Rolls

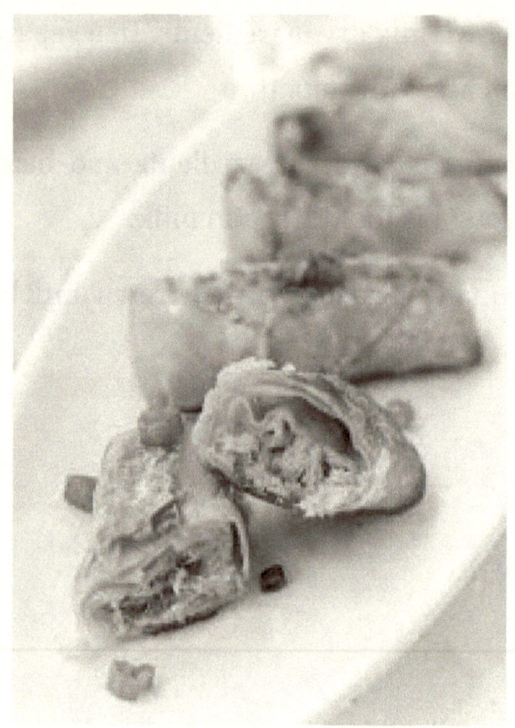

Preparation time: 10 minutes

Cooking time: 30 minutes

Servings: 12

Ingredients:

2 eggs

1 tbsp fat cream

79.38 g canned tuna canned (drained)

¼ chopped avocado

12 g lettuce

2 tbsp low carb mayonnaise (separate)

1 tsp chopped dill

1 tsp lemon juice

Sea salt and black pepper to taste

1 tsp butter

Direction

Break the eggs into a blender. Pour in heavy cream, and season with salt and pepper. Mix everything together until smooth.

Melt a teaspoon of oil in a medium pan. Gently pour the beaten eggs, cover and fry until tender.

Mix tuna, mayonnaise, dill and lemon juice in a bowl. Add salt and pepper and mix well.

Place the omelet on a plate and brush with mayonnaise. Layout a mixture of tuna, sliced avocado, and lettuce.

Roll up the omelet so that the filling is inside. Halve and serve warm with your favorite low-carb sauce.

Waffle Chicken Sandwich

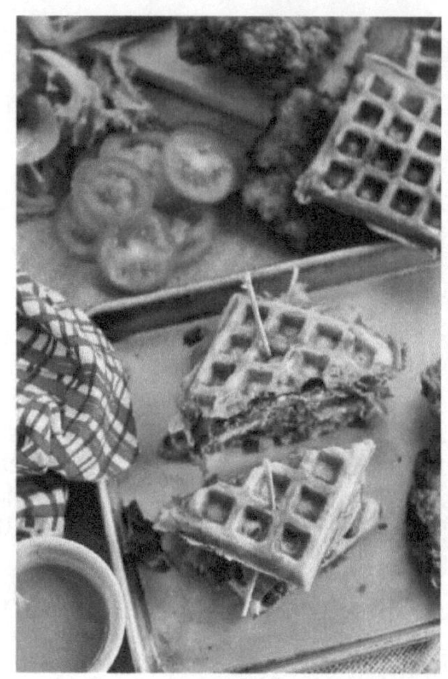

Preparation time: 10 minutes

Cooking time: 20 minutes

Servings: 12

Ingredients:

Waffles:

2 tbsp ghee

3 large eggs, protein separated from yolks

1/4 cup milk

1 cup almond flour

1/2 tsp salt

1 tsp vanilla

1 tbsp erythritis

A hen:

1 cup buttermilk (nonfat cream)

2 medium chicken breasts

1 large egg

Olive oil for frying

Salt and pepper to taste

1 tsp paprika

1/4 tsp cayenne powder

Additionally: maple syrup without sugar, bacon, pickles and mustard.

Direction

Cut the chicken breasts in half lengthwise. Cut these slices in half lengthwise, four strips into the chicken breast. Soak the buttermilk strips overnight.

Remove the chicken from buttermilk, then season with salt, pepper, cayenne powder and paprika.

In a bowl, beat the egg, then set the bowl aside. In a separate bowl, combine almond flour, as well as a little salt and pepper.

Lubricate each piece of chicken with an egg, then with almond flour. Grease each slice again with an egg and then with almond flour so that there are two layers of breading.

Heat a little olive oil in a pan, then quickly cook both sides of each chicken stripe so that it is fried outside. Put each piece of chicken on a baking sheet and cover with foil. Bake at 176 degrees for 15 minutes or until tender.

Preheat the waffle iron. Beat egg yolks, milk, erythritol, ghee, and vanilla together. Beat almond flour and salt until lumpy.

Beat the egg whites with a hand mixer until the foam is formed. Gently pour the eggs into the waffle dough, half at a time.

Lubricate the waffle iron, then add 1/3 cup serving of dough and cook each wafer for 5-6 minutes or until brown.

Serve wafers with chicken on top and mustard. Put a piece of bacon and two cucumbers on each wafer, then cover the sandwich with another waffle and sprinkle with sugar-free maple syrup. Poke a toothpick so that the sandwich does not fall apart before serving.

Carrot Cream Muffins

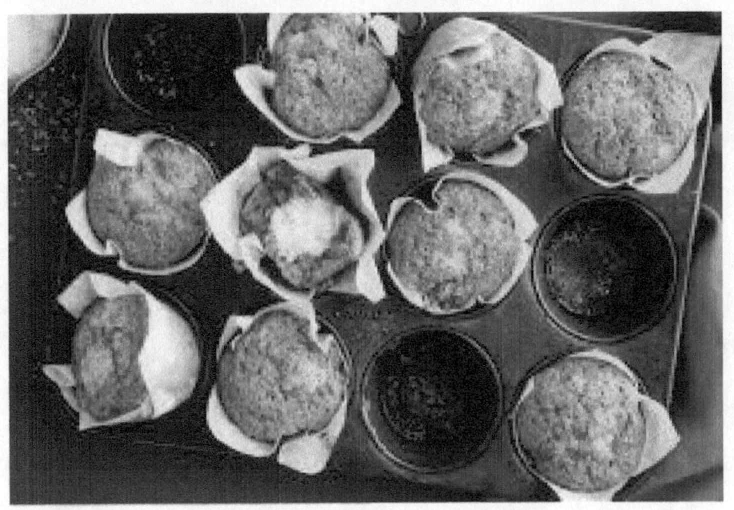

Preparation time: 10 minutes

Cooking time: 40 minutes

Servings: 12

Ingredients:

4 eggs (protein separated from yolks)

1 tsp greasy whipped cream

50 g of powdered erythritol

0.25 tsp stevia powder extract

56 g almond flour

60 g oat fiber

96 g carrots

0.5 tsp baking powder

62.5 g almond milk

56 g butter

1 tsp allspice

1 tsp cinnamon

24.75 g chopped pecans

Filling:

226.8 g cream cheese

1 egg

1 tbsp coconut flour

50 g of powdered erythritol

0.25 tsp stevia powder extract

0.5 tsp vanilla extract

Direction

Beat egg white and cream until foamy.

In a separate bowl, combine egg yolks, erythritol, stevia, almond flour, oat fiber, almond milk, butter, allspice, cinnamon and carrots until smooth.

Gently add egg white and pecans.

Pour the batter into a well-greased muffin pan.

Filling:

Beat cream cheese with egg, coconut flour, 1/4 cup erythritol, 1/4 teaspoon of stevia and 1/2 teaspoon of vanilla until a homogeneous mass is formed.

Put a couple of teaspoons of the toppings on each muffin.

Bake at 176 degrees for 20-25 minutes.

Chia Seed Pumpkin Pudding

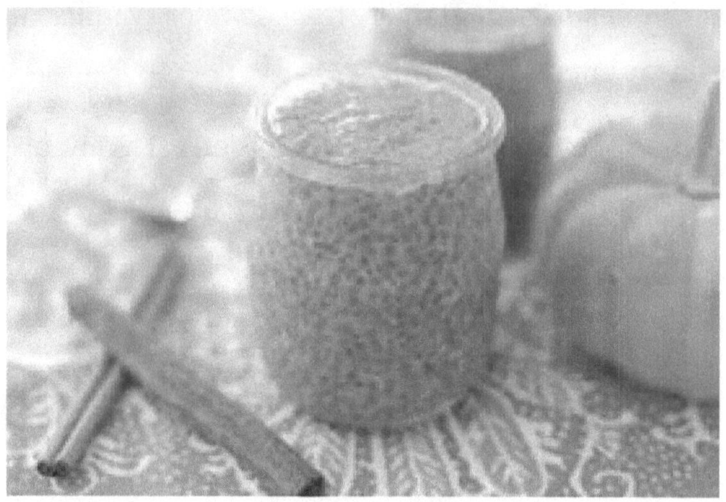

Preparation time: 10 minutes

Cooking time: 30 minutes

Servings: 12

Ingredients:

339 g coconut milk or unsweetened almond milk

184 g pumpkin puree

12 drops of liquid stevia

1 tsp vanilla extract

0.5 tsp cinnamon

0.25 tsp ground ginger

0.25 tsp nutmeg

0.13 tsp carnations

42.5 g chia seeds

Direction

Beat milk, pumpkin, vanilla, and spices together. Add chia seeds and mix.

Refrigerate for a couple of hours or overnight.

Matcha Chia Seed Pudding

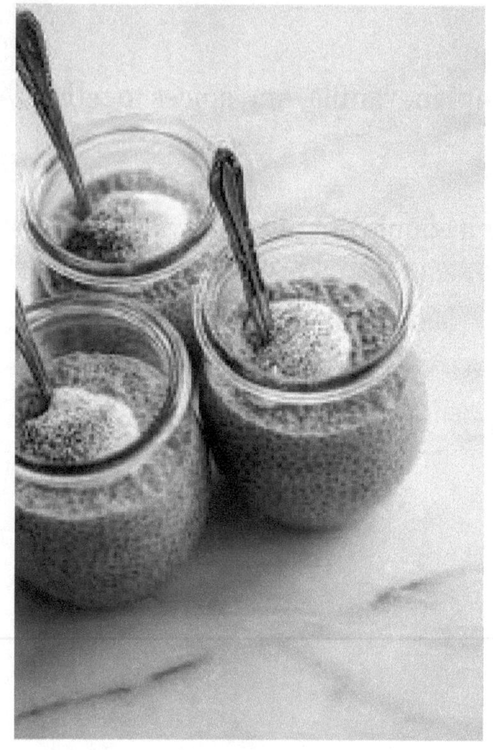

Preparation time: 10 minutes

Cooking time: 20 minutes

Servings: 12

Ingredients:

4 matcha green tea bags

83.33 ml of boiling water

45.5 g low carbohydrate sweetener

437.5 ml unsweetened almond or coconut milk

56.67 g chia seeds

Direction

Brew green tea for about 3-5 minutes. Take out the bags.

Add sweetener, almond milk and chia seeds to brewed tea. Mix well.

Continue stirring every 5 minutes for 15 minutes.

Serve and cool.

Pepperoni Cheese Muffins

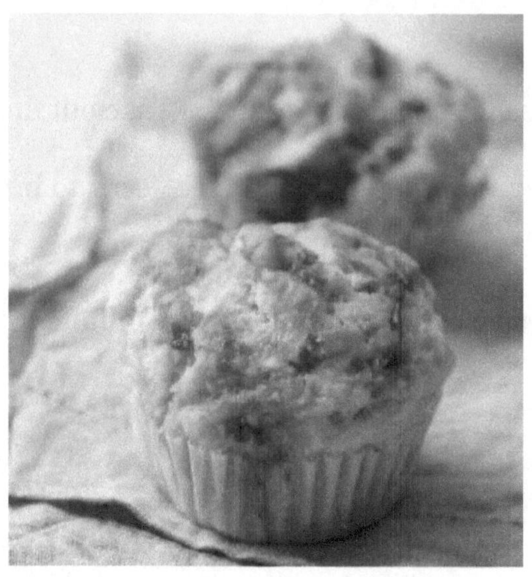

Preparation time: 10 minutes

Cooking time: 40 minutes

Servings: 12

Ingredients:

141.75 g cream cheese

50 g minced Parmesan cheese

30 g coconut flour

74.67 g almond flour

1 tsp baking powder

0.5 tsp salt

3 tbsp water

5 beaten eggs

56.5 g mini pepperoni

112 g chopped mozzarella

Direction

Preheat the oven to 204 ° C. Lubricate the muffin tins.

In a large bowl, combine cream cheese, grated Parmesan cheese, almond and coconut flour, baking powder, salt, water, and beaten eggs.

Add pepperoni and 1/2 cup mozzarella cheese.

Fill the muffin molds 1/2 to 3/4.

Top with 1/2 cup mozzarella cheese.

Bake for 25-30 minutes, or until the muffins are firm and lightly browned.

Cheese and Egg Tart

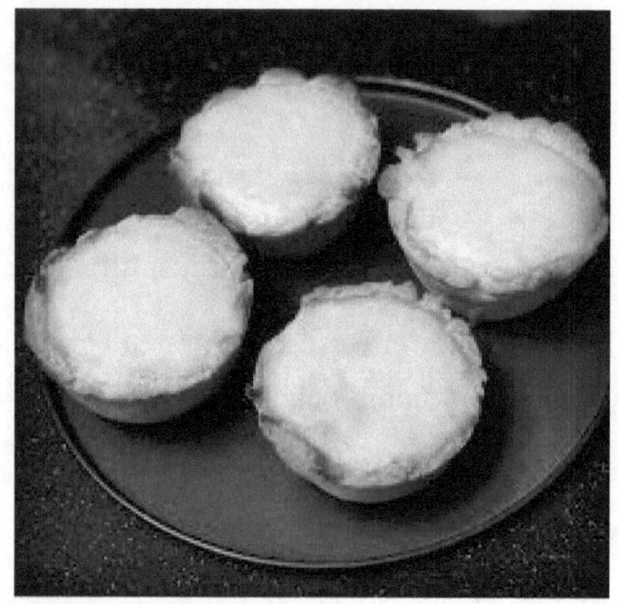

Preparation time: 10 minutes

Cooking time: 30 minutes

Servings: 12

Ingredients:

227 g grated cheddar cheese

12 large eggs

114 g soft cream cheese

12 tablespoons unsalted melted butter

Salt and pepper to taste

Direction

Put about half the cheese in a 9.5-inch cake pan.

Add eggs and cream cheese to a food processor or blender.

Beat eggs and cream cheese by slowly adding melted butter.

Pour the egg mixture onto the cheese in a baking pan.

Sprinkle the remaining grated cheese on top.

Bake at 162 ° C for 45 minutes.

Remove from the oven and cool on the wire rack for several minutes before slicing.

Store leftovers in the refrigerator (about a week) or in the freezer (for a longer period).

Low carb muesli

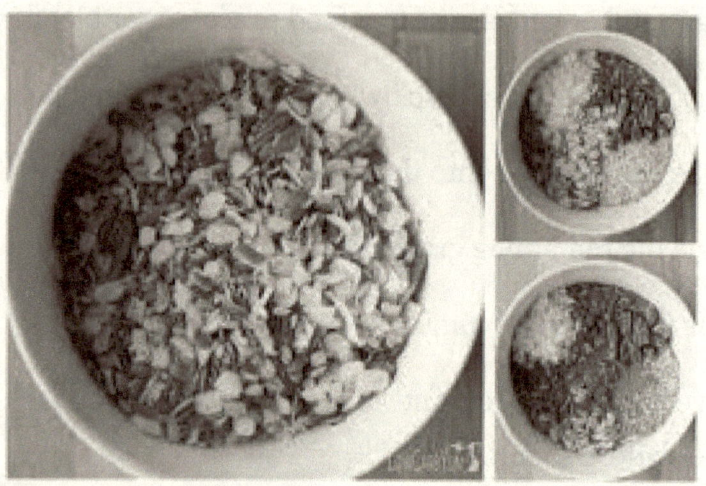

Preparation time: 10 minutes

Cooking time: 40 minutes

Servings: 12

Ingredients:

134 g of sunflower seeds

85 g unsweetened coconut

64 g pumpkin seeds

143 g chopped almonds

49.5 g pecans

100 g hemp seeds

2 tsp cinnamon

0.5 tsp vanilla extract

0.25 tsp liquid stevia

Direction

Thoroughly mix all the ingredients in a large bowl.

Place on a baking tray and bake at a temperature of 176 degrees for about 7-8 minutes.

Let cool. Store in an airtight container.

Each serving is about 1/3 cup. It goes well with almond milk!

Garlic Cauliflower Fried Rice

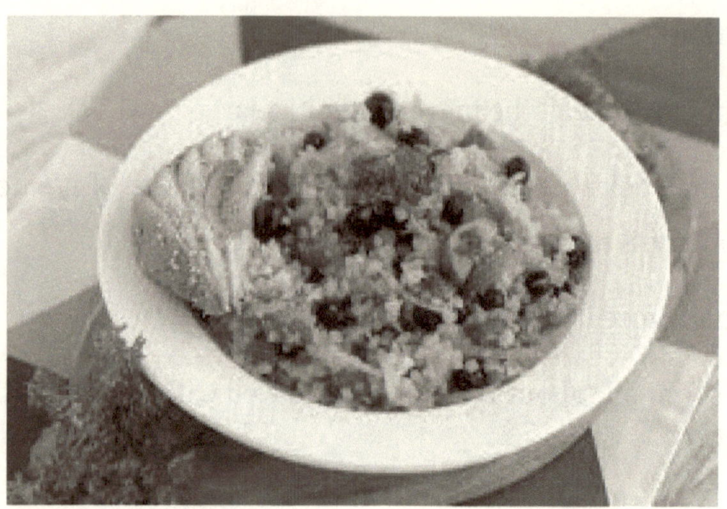

Preparation time: 10 minutes

Cooking time: 30 minutes

Servings: 12

Ingredients:

3 tbsp olive oil

3-4 minced garlic cloves

480 g cooked cauliflower

3 eggs whipped with a fork (optional)

2 tbsp unsweetened almond milk

3 slices of ham or bacon

1 tbsp soy sauce

Chopped onion (optional)

Direction

Heat the olive oil over medium heat in a large skillet.

Add the garlic (and chopped onions when using) and simmer until the garlic begins to brown.

Add the cauliflower and mix, then slide aside.

Mix eggs and almond milk, then pour onto another pan and fry the omelet.

Add scrambled eggs to cauliflower and mix. Add the ham.

Mix with soy sauce and stir over medium heat for a minute or two until everything is warm.

Bacon Egg Muffins

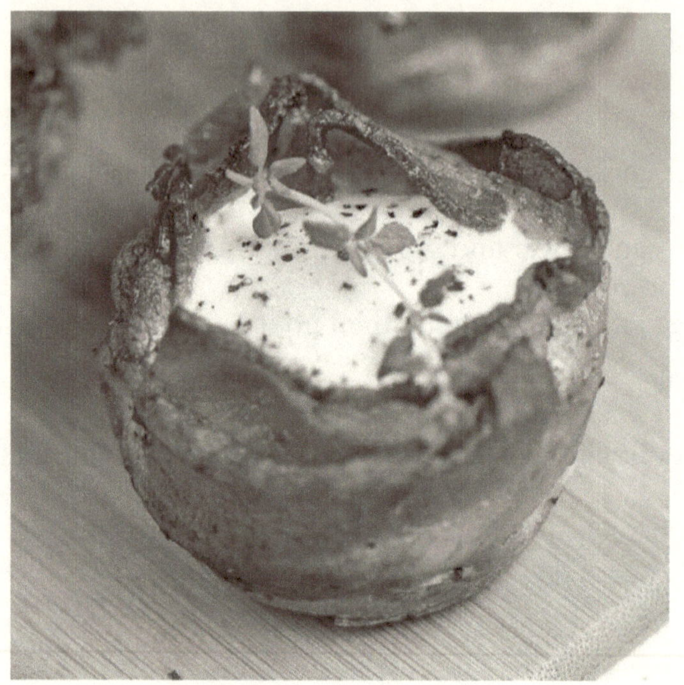

Preparation time: 10 minutes

Cooking time: 40 minutes

Servings: 12

Ingredients:

12 slices of bacon

12 large eggs

226 g grated cheddar cheese

Direction

Bake bacon in the oven at 204 ° C for 10-12 minutes. Take it out before it becomes crispy.

Sprinkle cupcake tins (12 pcs.) With a nonstick spray. Layout each bacon pan.

Beat the eggs and add the grated cheese.

Spread the mixture over the tins.

Bake for about 25 minutes at 176 ° C.

Chapter 6: Lunch

Herb Spaghetti Squash

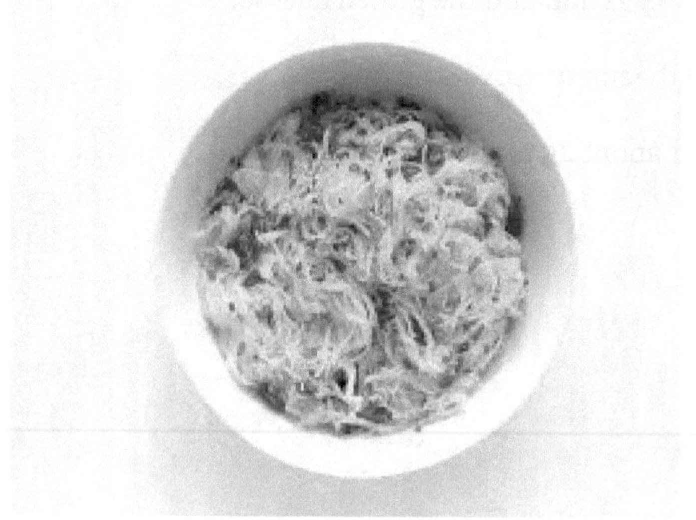

Preparation time: minutes

Servings: 4

Ingredients:

4 cups spaghetti squash, cooked

½ tsp pepper

½ tsp sage

1 tsp dried parsley

1 tsp dried thyme

1 tsp dried rosemary

1 tsp garlic powder

2 tbsp olive oil

1 tsp salt

Directions:

Preheat the oven to 350 F/ 180 C.

Add all ingredients into the mixing bowl and mix well to combine.

Transfer bowl mixture to the oven safe dish and cook in preheated oven for 15 minutes.

Stir well and serve.

Delicious Cabbage Steaks

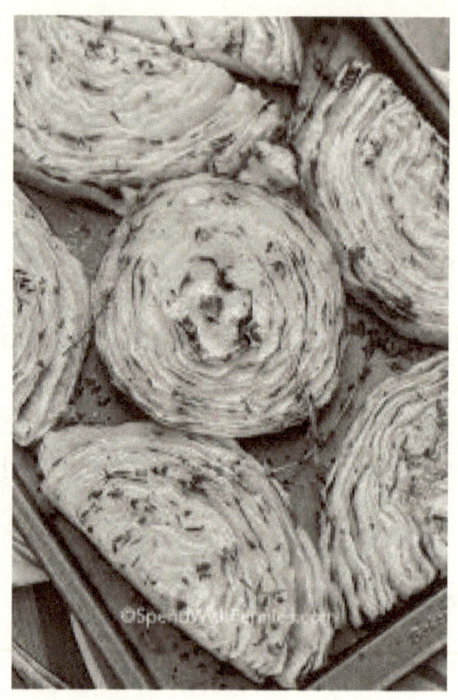

Preparation time: 1 hour 10 minutes

Servings: 6

Ingredients:

1 medium cabbage head, slice 1" thick

2 tbsp olive oil

1 tbsp garlic, minced

Pepper

Salt

Directions:

In a small bowl, mix together garlic and olive oil.

Brush garlic and olive oil mixture onto both sides of sliced cabbage.

Season cabbage slices with pepper and salt.

Place cabbage slices onto a baking tray and bake at 350 F/ 180 C for 1 hour. Turn after 30 minutes.

Serve and enjoy.

Mexican Cauliflower Rice

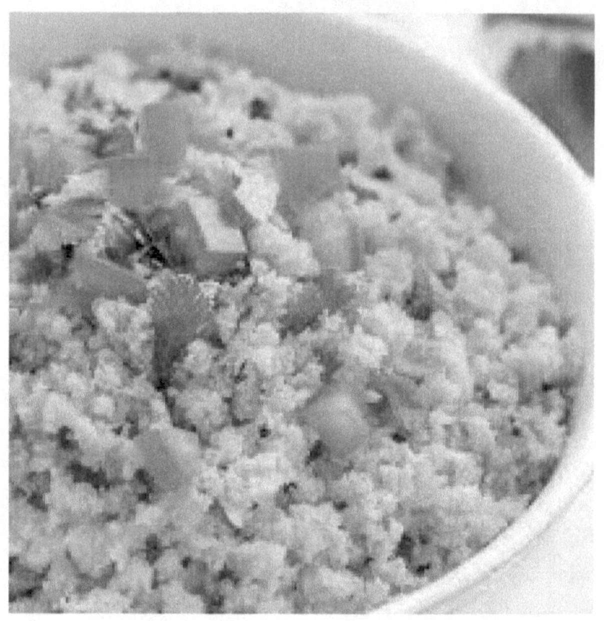

Preparation time: 25 minutes

Servings: 4

Ingredients:

1 medium cauliflower head, cut into florets

½ cup tomato sauce

¼ tsp black pepper

1 tsp chili powder

2 garlic cloves, minced

½ medium onion, diced

1 tbsp coconut oil

½ tsp sea sal

Directions:

Add cauliflower florets into the food processor and process until it looks like rice.

Heat oil in a pan over medium-high heat.

Add onion to the pan and sauté for 5 minutes or until softened.

Add garlic and cook for 1 minute.

Add cauliflower rice, chili powder, pepper, and salt. Stir well.

Add tomato sauce and cook for 5 minutes.

Stir well and serve warm.

Asparagus Mash

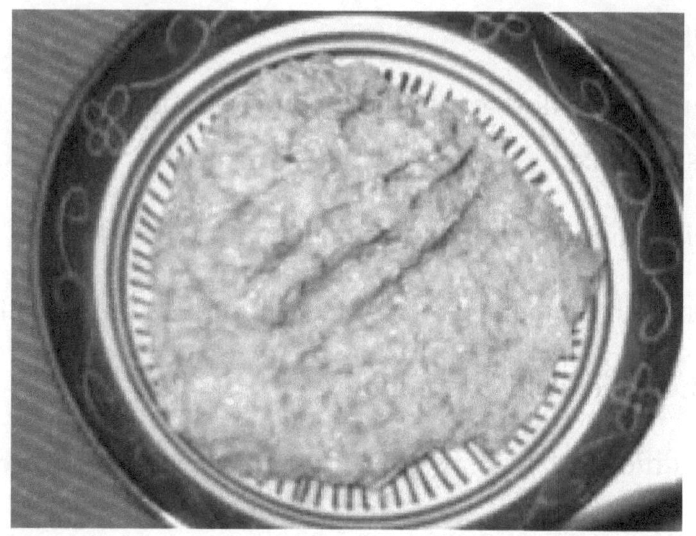

Preparation time: 20 minutes

Servings: 2

Ingredients:

10 asparagus shoots, chopped

1 tsp lemon juice

2 tbsp fresh parsley

2 tbsp coconut cream

1 small onion, diced

1 tbsp coconut oil

Pepper

Salt

Directions:

Sauté onion in coconut oil until onion is softened.

Blanch chopped asparagus in hot water for 2 minutes and drain immediately.

Add sautéed onion, lemon juice, parsley, coconut cream, asparagus, pepper, and salt into the blender and blend until smooth.

Serve warm and enjoy.

Creamy Squash Soup

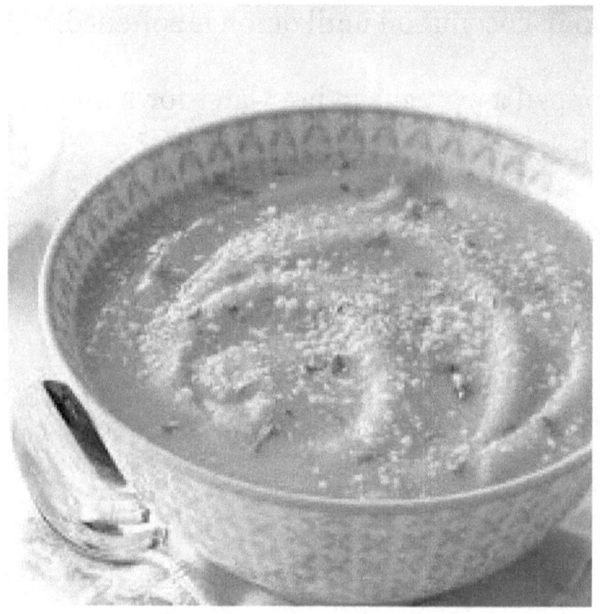

Preparation time: 35 minutes

Servings: 8

Ingredients:

3 cups butternut squash, chopped

1 ½ cups unsweetened coconut milk

1 tbsp coconut oil

1 tsp dried onion flakes

1 tbsp curry powder

4 cups water

1 garlic clove

1 tsp kosher salt

Directions:

Add squash, coconut oil, onion flakes, curry powder, water, garlic, and salt into a large saucepan. Bring to boil over high heat.

Turn heat to medium and simmer for 20 minutes.

Puree the soup using a blender until smooth. Return soup to the saucepan and stir in coconut milk and cook for 2 minutes.

Stir well and serve hot.

Spinach with Coconut Milk

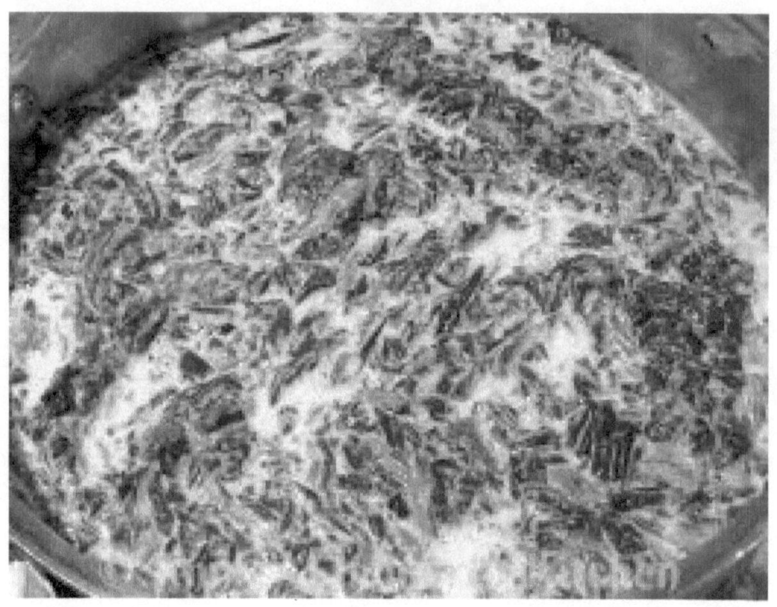

Preparation time: 25 minutes

Servings: 6

Ingredients:

16 oz spinach

2 tsp curry powder

13.5 oz coconut milk

1 tsp lemon zest

½ tsp salt

Directions:

Add spinach in pan and heat over medium heat. Once it is hot then add curry paste and few tablespoons of coconut milk. Stir well.

Add remaining coconut milk, lemon zest, and salt and cook until thickened.

Serve and enjoy.

Sautéed Brussels sprouts

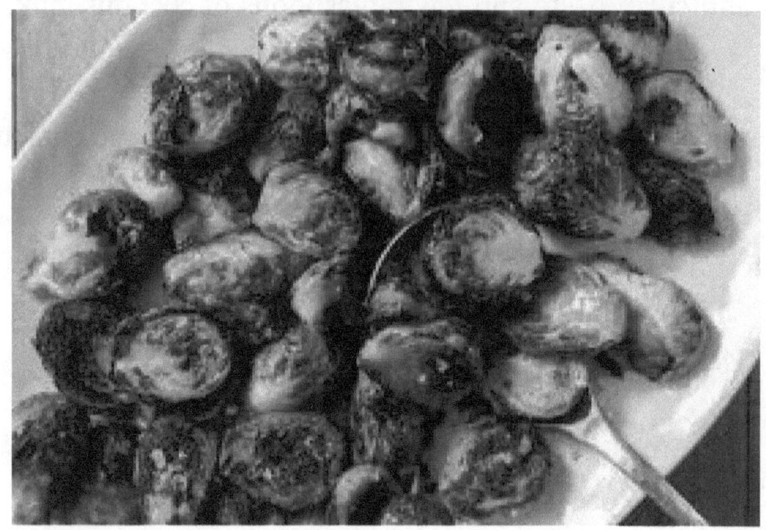

Preparation time: 25 minutes

Servings: 6

Ingredients:

2 lbs Brussels sprouts, remove stems and shred Brussels sprouts

2 oz onion, minced

3 garlic cloves, minced

1 1/2 tbsp olive oil

Pepper

Salt

Directions:

Heat olive oil in a pan over medium heat.

Add onion and garlic and sauté for 5 minutes.

Add Brussels sprouts and sauté over medium-high heat for 5-7 minutes. Season with pepper and salt.

Serve and enjoy.

Turnip Carrot Salad

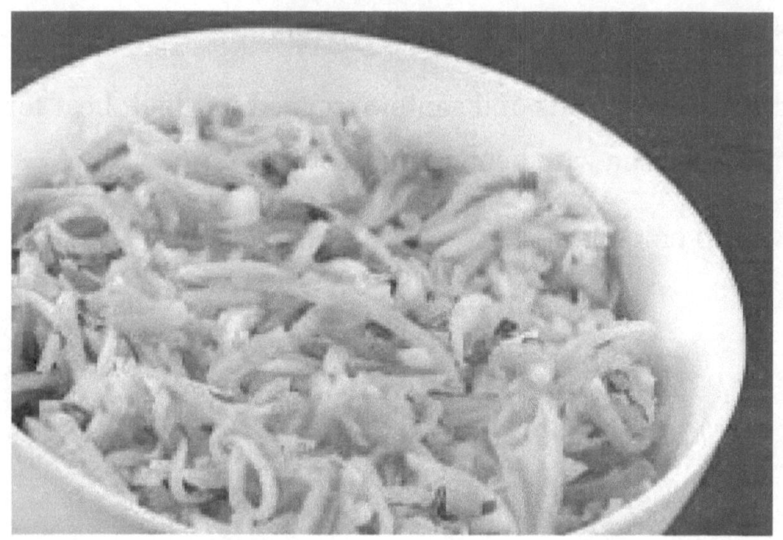

Preparation time: 50 minutes

Servings: 4

Ingredients:

1 turnip, shredded

1/4 tsp dill

3 cups cabbage, shredded

1 carrot, shredded

1 green pepper, chopped

1 tsp salt

Directions:

Add cabbage and salt in a bowl. Cover bowl and set aside for 40 minutes.

Wash and cabbage and dry well.

Add cabbage in a bowl with remaining ingredients and toss well.

Serve and enjoy.

Baked Asparagus

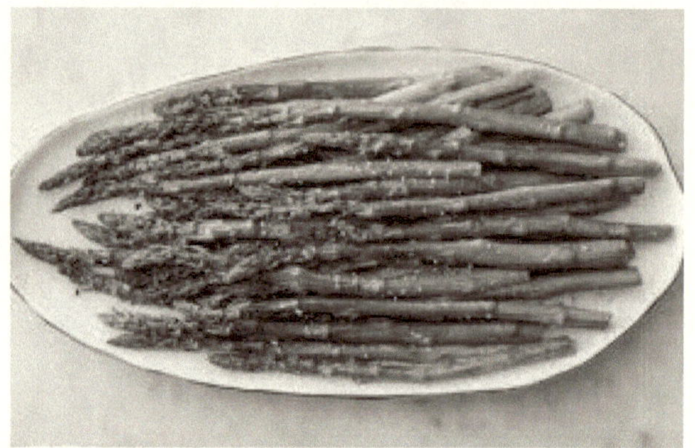

Preparation time: 25 minutes

Servings: 4

Ingredients:

40 asparagus spears

2 tbsp vegetable seasoning

2 tbsp garlic powder

2 tbsp salt

Directions:

Preheat the oven to 450 F/ 232 C.

Arrange all asparagus spears on baking tray and season with vegetable seasoning, garlic powder, and salt.

Place in preheated oven and bake for 20 minutes.

Serve warm and enjoy.

Avocado Mint Soup

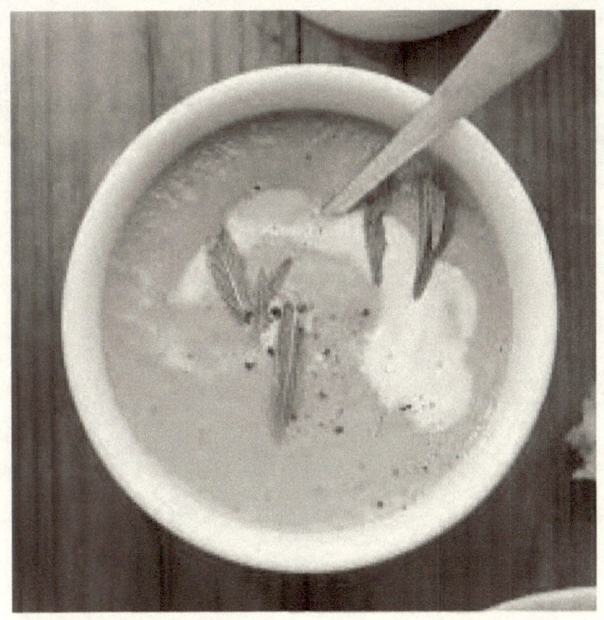

Preparation time: 10 minutes

Servings: 2

Ingredients:

1 medium avocado, peeled, pitted, and cut into pieces

1 cup coconut milk

2 romaine lettuce leaves

20 fresh mint leaves

1 tbsp fresh lime juice

1/8 tsp salt

Directions:

Add all ingredients into the blender and blend until smooth. Soup should be thick not as a puree.

Pour into the serving bowls and place in the refrigerator for 10 minutes.

Stir well and serve chilled.

Vegetable Salad

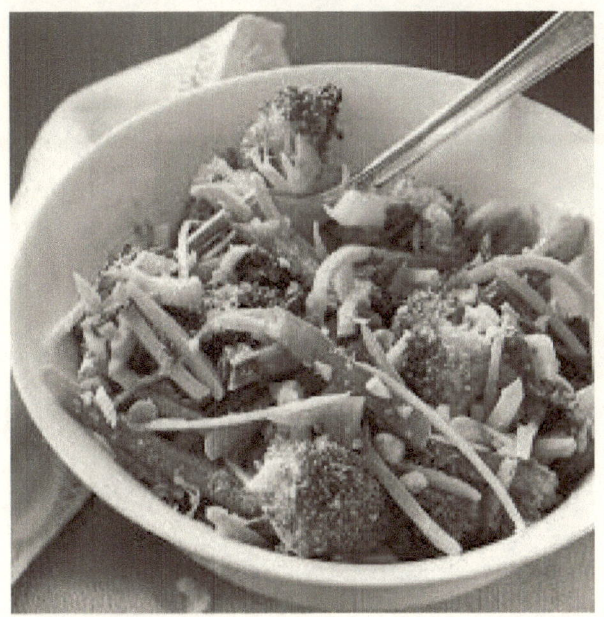

Preparation time: 15 minutes

Servings: 6

Ingredients:

2 cups cauliflower florets

2 cups carrots, chopped

2 cups cherry tomatoes, halved

2 tbsp shallots, minced

1 bell pepper, seeded and chopped

1 cucumber, seeded and chopped

For dressing:

2 garlic cloves, minced

1/2 cup red wine vinegar

1/2 cup olive oil

Pepper

Sal

Directions:

In a small bowl, combine together all dressing ingredients.

Add all salad ingredients to the large bowl and toss well.

Pour dressing over salad and toss well.

Place salad bowl in refrigerator for 4 hours.

Serve chilled and enjoy.

Lemon Zucchini Noodles

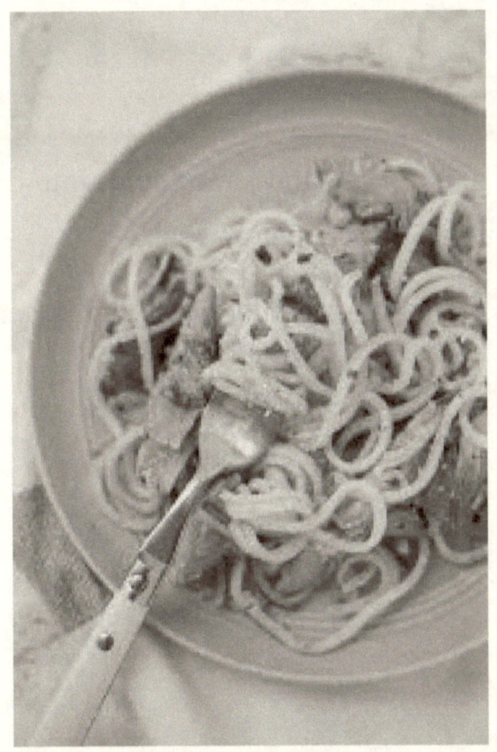

Preparation time: 15 minutes

Servings: 4

Ingredients:

4 small zucchini, spiralized into noodles

2 garlic cloves

2 cups fresh basil leaves

2 tsp lemon juice

1/3 cup olive oil

Pepper

Salt

Directions:

Add garlic, basil, olive oil, and lemon juice into the blender and blend well. Season with pepper and salt.

In a large bowl, combine together pesto and zucchini noodles.

Stir well and serve.

Classic Cabbage Slaw

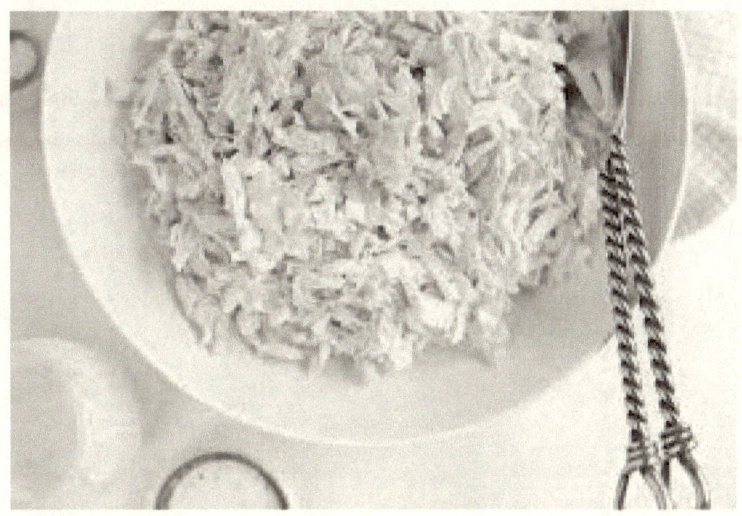

Preparation time: 20 minutes

Servings: 3

Ingredients:

4 cups green cabbage, shredded

2 garlic cloves

1 tbsp sesame oil

2 tbsp tamari

1 tsp vinegar

1 tsp chili paste

½ cup macadamia nuts, chopped

Directions:

Toss shredded green cabbage in a pan with chili paste, sesame oil, vinegar, and tamari on medium-low heat.

Add garlic and cook for 5 minutes or until cabbage is softened.

Stir everything well. Add macadamia nuts and cook for 5 minutes.

Stir well and serve.

Delicious Herb Cauliflower Rice

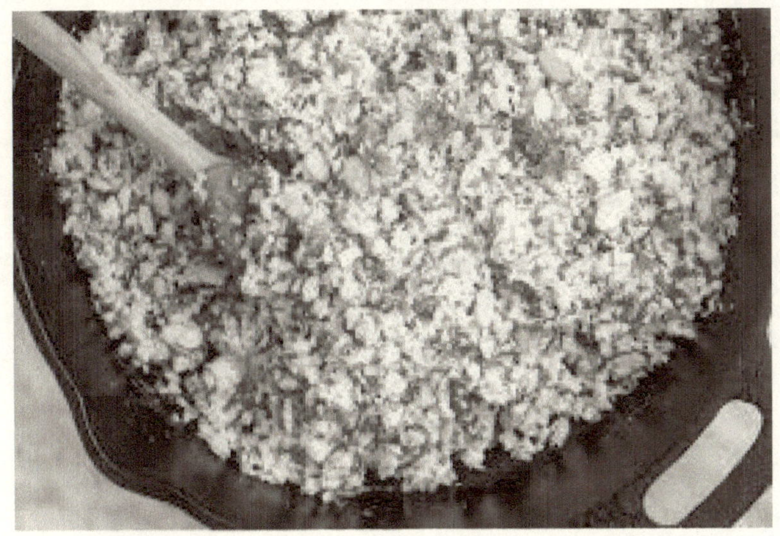

Preparation time: 20 minutes

Servings: 3

Ingredients:

10 oz cauliflower rice

4 oz mushrooms, sliced

8 oz asparagus, cut into 3" pieces

1/2 tsp rosemary

1/2 tsp cayenne

2 tbsp olive oil

6 baby carrots, sliced

1/2 tsp black pepper

1/2 tsp sea salt

Directions:

Heat olive oil in a pan over medium heat.

Add vegetables to a pan and sauté for 3-4 minutes.

Add cauliflower rice and spices and sauté for 10 minutes.

Serve and enjoy.

Mushroom Asparagus

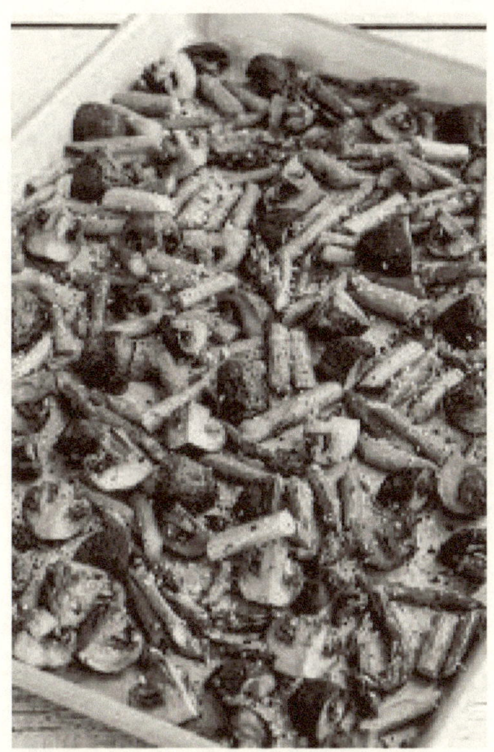

Preparation time: 10 minutes

Servings: 4

Ingredients:

1 lb asparagus, trimmed and cut into pieces

1/4 cup water

12 mushrooms, sliced

3 tbsp olive oil

Pepper

Salt

Directions:

Heat oil in a large pan over medium heat.

Add mushroom and salt and sauté for 1 minute or until mushroom is golden brown.

Remove mushrooms to plate and add asparagus season with pepper and salt.

Cook asparagus for 2 minutes or until softened.

Remove from heat and mix with mushrooms.

Serve and enjoy.

Tomato Eggplant Spinach Salad

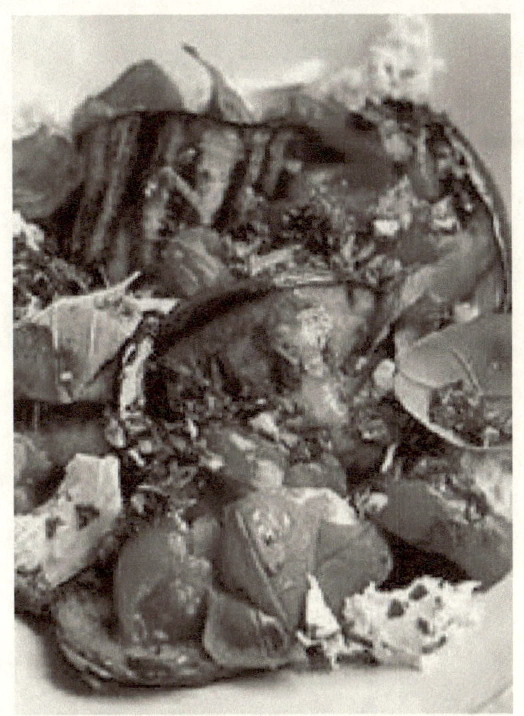

Preparation time: 30 minutes

Servings: 4

Ingredients:

1 large eggplant, cut into 3/4 inch slices

5 oz spinach

1 tbsp sun-dried tomatoes, chopped

1 tbsp oregano, chopped

1 tbsp parsley, chopped

1 tbsp fresh mint, chopped

1 tbsp shallot, chopped

For dressing:

1/4 cup olive oil

1/2 lemon juice

1/2 tsp smoked paprika

1 tsp Dijon mustard

1 tsp tahini

2 garlic cloves, minced

Pepper

Salt

Directions:

Place sliced eggplants into the large bowl and sprinkle with salt and set aside for minutes.

In a small bowl mix together all dressing ingredients. Set aside.

Heat grill to medium-high heat.

In a large bowl, add shallot, sun-dried tomatoes, herbs, and spinach.

Rinse eggplant slices and pat dry with paper towel.

Brush eggplant slices with olive oil and grill on medium high heat for 3-4 minutes on each side.

Let cool the grilled eggplant slices then cut into quarters.

Add eggplant to the salad bowl and pour dressing over salad. Toss well.

Serve and enjoy.

Roasted Cauliflower

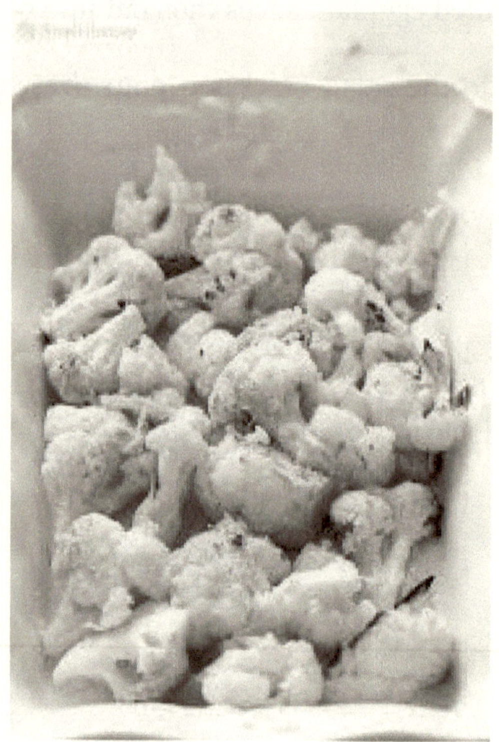

Preparation time: 20 minutes

Servings: 4

Ingredients:

1 large caul iflower head, cut into florets

1 lemon zest

3 tbsp olive oil

2 tsp lemon juice

½ tsp Italian seasoning

½ tsp garlic powder

¼ tsp pepper

¼ tsp salt

Directions:

Preheat the oven to 425 F/ 218 C.

In a bowl, combine together olive oil, lemon juice, Italian seasoning, garlic powder, lemon zest, pepper, and salt.

Add cauliflower florets to the bowl and toss well.

Spread cauliflower florets on baking tray and roast in preheated oven for 15 minutes.

Serve and enjoy.

Cauliflower Coconut Rice

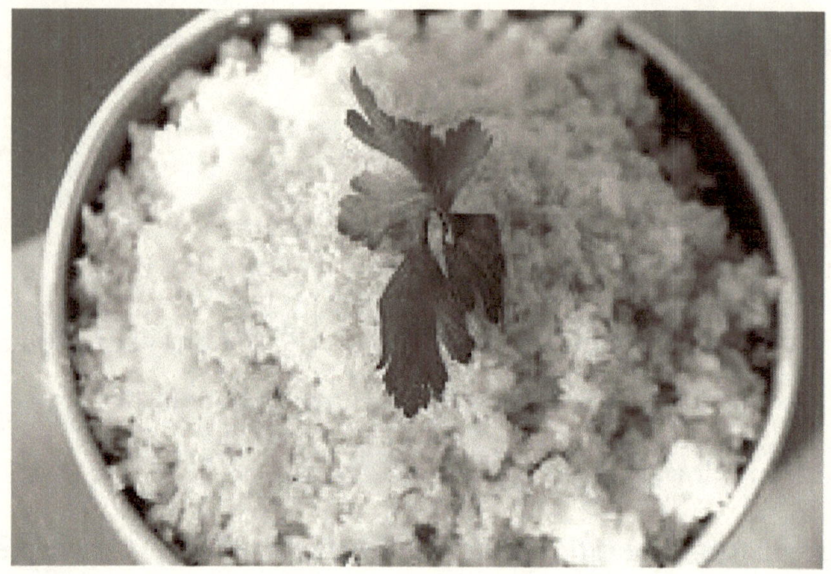

Preparation time: 20 minutes

Servings: 3

Ingredients:

3 cups cauliflower rice

½ tsp onion powder

1 tsp chili paste

2/3 cup coconut milk

Salt

Directions:

Add all ingredients to the pan and heat over medium-low heat. Stir to combine.

Cook for 10 minutes. Stir after every 2 minutes.

Remove lid and cook until excess liquid absorbed.

Serve and enjoy.

Ginger Avocado Kale Salad

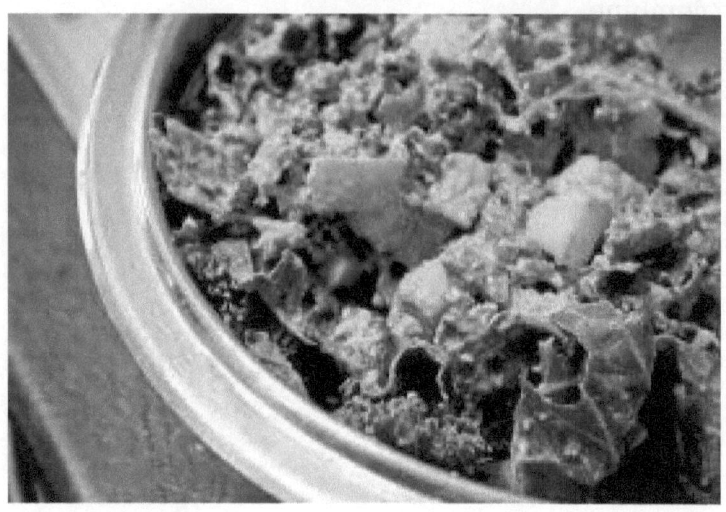

Preparation time: 15 minutes

Servings: 4

Ingredients:

1 avocado, peeled and sliced

1 tbsp ginger, grated

1/2 lb kale, chopped

1/4 cup parsley, chopped

2 fresh scallions, chopped

Directions:

Add all ingredients into the mixing bowl and toss well.

Serve and enjoy.

Refreshing Cucumber Salad

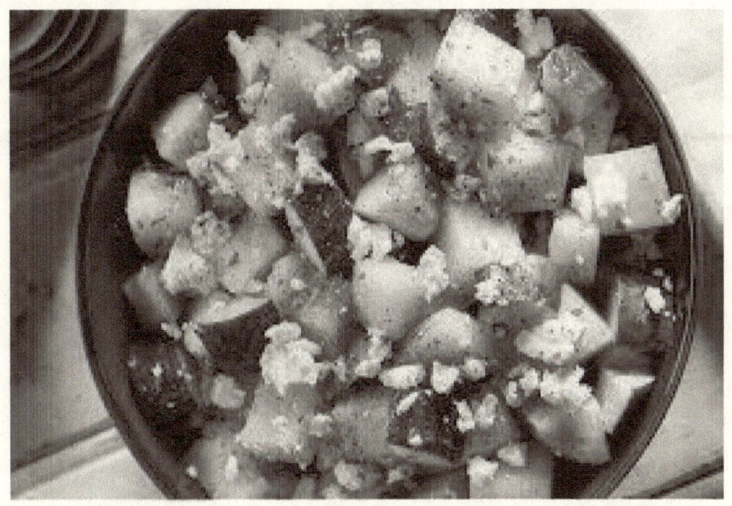

Preparation time: 10 minutes

Servings: 4

Ingredients:

1/3 cup cucumber basil ranch

1 cucumber, chopped

3 tomatoes, chopped

3 tbsp fresh herbs, chopped

½ onion, sliced

Directions:

Add all ingredients into the large mixing bowl and toss well.

Serve immediately and enjoy.

Cabbage Coconut Salad

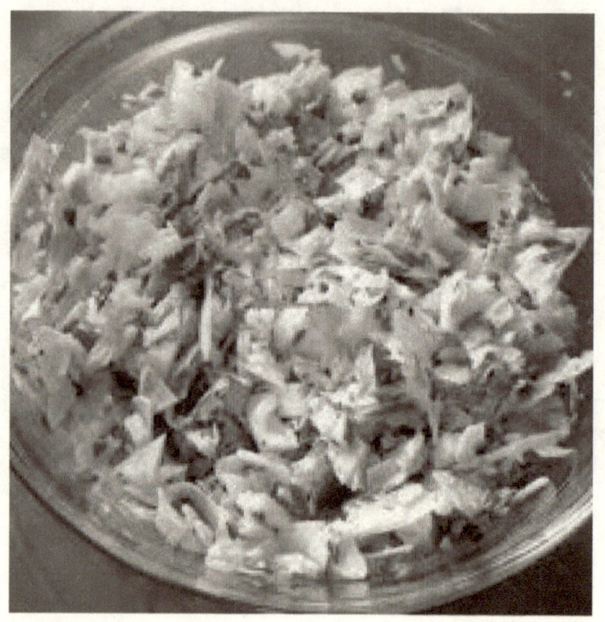

Preparation time: 15 minutes

Servings: 4

Ingredients:

1/3 cup unsweetened desiccated coconut

½ medium head cabbage, shredded

2 tsp sesame seeds

¼ cup tamari sauce

¼ cup olive oil

1 fresh lemon juice

½ tsp cumin

½ tsp curry powder

½ tsp ginger powder

Directions:

Add all ingredients into the large mixing bowl and toss well.

Place salad bowl in refrigerator for 1 hour.

Serve and enjoy.

Avocado Cabbage Salad

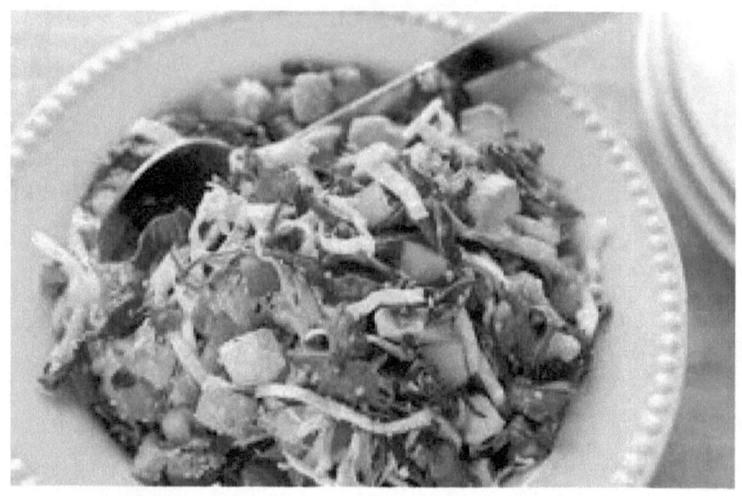

Preparation time: 20 minutes

Servings: 4

Ingredients:

2 avocados, diced

4 cups cabbage, shredded

3 tbsp fresh par sley, chopped

2 tbsp apple cider vinegar

4 tbsp olive oil

1 cup cherry tomatoes, halved

1/2 tsp pepper

1 1/2 tsp sea salt

Directions:

Add cabbage, avocados, and tomatoes to a medium bowl and mix well.

In a small bowl, whisk together oil, parsley, vinegar, pepper, and salt.

Pour dressing over vegetables and mix well.

Serve and enjoy.

Turnip Salad

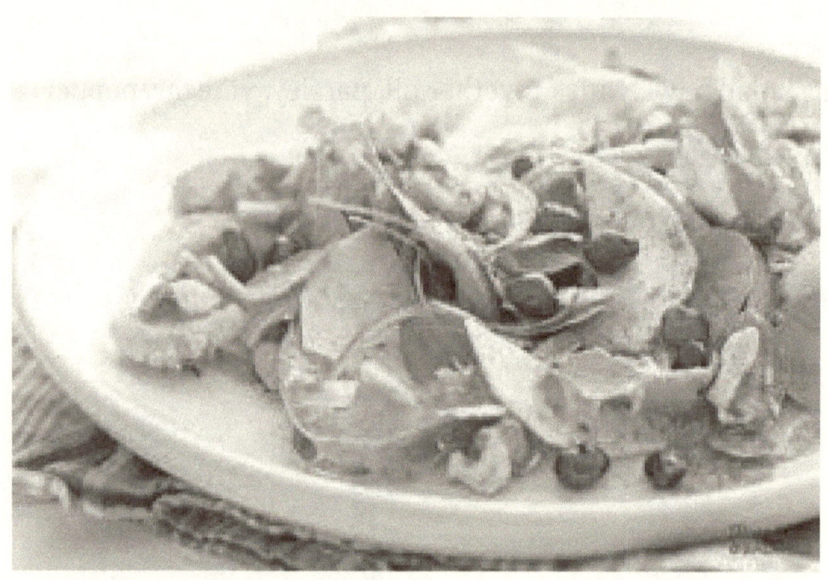

Preparation time: 10 minutes

Servings: 4

Ingredients:

4 white turnips, spiralized

1 lemon juice

4 dill sprigs, chopped

2 tbsp olive oil

1 1/2 tsp salt

Directions:

Season spiralized turnip with salt and gently massage with hands.

Add lemon juice and dill. Season with pepper and salt.

Drizzle with olive oil and combine everything well.

Serve immediately and enjoy.

Roasted Almond Broccoli

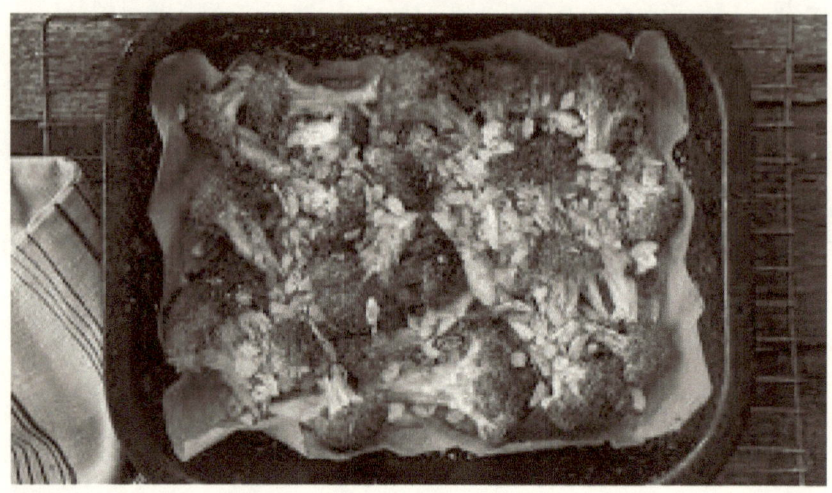

Preparation time: 25 minutes

Servings: 4

Ingredients:

1 1/2 lbs broccoli florets

3 tbsp olive oil

1 tbsp fresh lemon juice

3 tbsp slivered almonds, toasted

2 garlic cloves, sliced

1/4 tsp pepper

1/4 tsp salt

Directions:

Preheat the oven to 425 F/ 218 C.

Spray baking dish with cooking spray.

Add broccoli, pepper, salt, garlic, and oil in large bowl and toss well.

Spread broccoli on the prepared baking dish and roast in preheated oven for 20 minutes.

Add lemon juice and almonds over broccoli and toss well.

Serve and enjoy.

Creamy Garlic Onion Soup

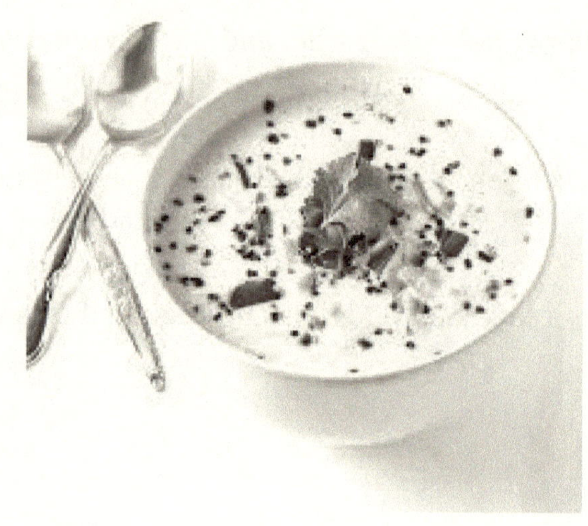

Preparation time: 45 minutes

Servings: 4

Ingredients:

1 onion, sliced

4 cups vegetable stock

1 1/2 tbsp olive oil

1 shallot, sliced

2 garlic clove, chopped

1 leek, sliced

Salt

Directions:

Add stock and olive oil in a saucepan and bring to boil.

Add remaining ingredients and stir well.

Cover and simmer for 25 minutes.

Puree the soup using an immersion blender until smooth.

Stir well and serve warm.

Cauliflower Spinach Soup

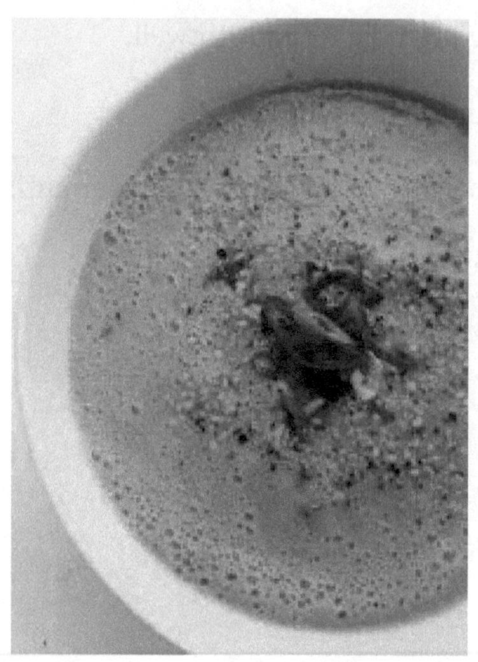

Preparation time: 45 minutes

Servings: 5

Ingredients:

1/2 cup unsweetened coconut milk

5 oz fresh spinac h, chopped

5 watercress, chopped

8 cups vegetable stock

1 lb cauliflower, chopped

Salt

Directions:

Add stock and cauliflower in a large saucepan and bring to boil over medium heat for 15 minutes.

Add spinach and watercress and cook for another 10 minutes.

Remove from heat and puree the soup using a blender until smooth.

Add coconut milk and stir well. Season with salt.

Stir well and serve hot.

Coconut Curry

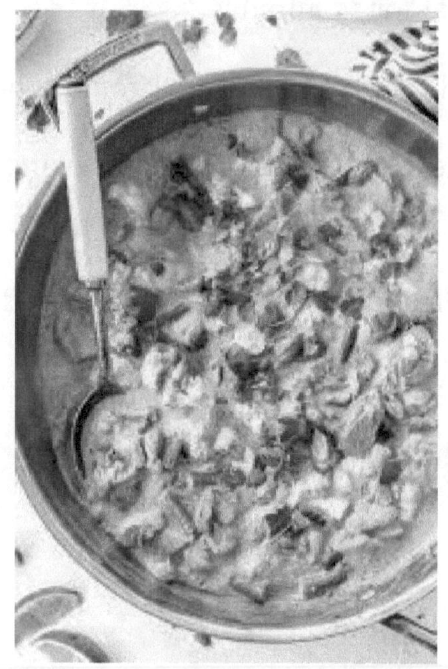

Preparation time: 30 minutes

Servings: 4

Ingredients:

1/2 cup coconut cream

1/4 medium onion, sliced

2 tsp soy sauce

1 tsp ginger, minced

1 tsp garlic, minced

4 tbsp coconut oil

2 cups spinach

1 cup broccoli florets

1 tbsp red curry past

Directions:

Heat coconut oil in a saucepan over medium-high heat.

Add onion in a pan and cook until softened. Add garlic sauté for a minute.

Turn heat to medium-low and add broccoli and stir well.

Once broccoli is cooked then add curry paste and stir for 1 minute.

Add spinach over the top of broccoli and cook until wilted.

Add ginger, soy sauce, and coconut cream and stir well. Simmer for 10 minutes.

Stir well and serve.

Spicy Broccoli

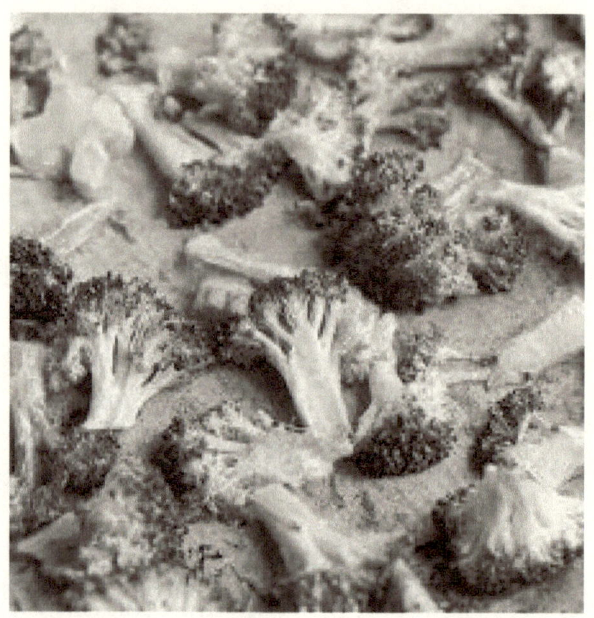

Preparation time: 25 minutes

Servings: 5

Ingredients:

2 tbsp fresh ginger, grated

2 tsp chili pepper, chopped

8 cups broccoli florets

1/2 cup olive oil

2 fresh lime juice

4 garlic cloves, chopped

Directions:

Add broccoli florets into the steamer and steam for 8 minutes.

Meanwhile, for dressing in a small bowl, combine together lime juice, oil, ginger, garlic, and chili pepper.

Add steamed broccoli in a large mixing bowl then pour dressing over broccoli. Toss well.

Serve and enjoy.

Tomato Pumpkin Soup

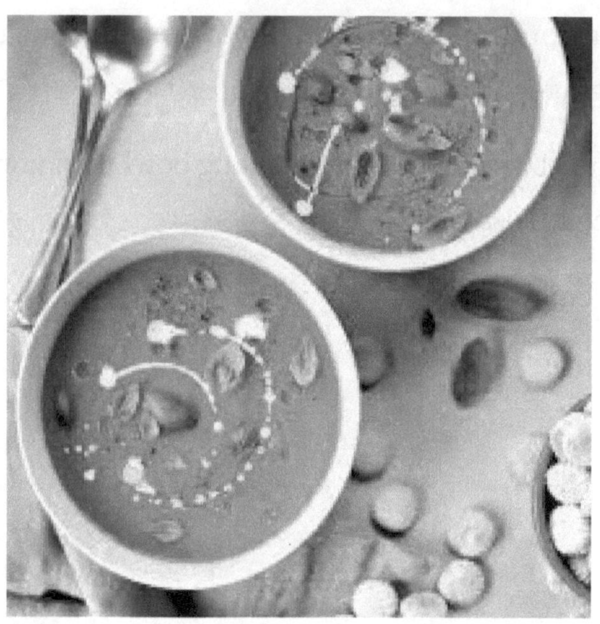

Preparation time: 25 minutes

Servings: 4

Ingredients:

2 cups pumpkin, diced

1/2 cup tomato, chopped

1/2 cup onion, chopped

1 1/2 tsp curry powder

1/2 tsp paprika

2 cups vegetable stock

1 tsp olive oil

1/2 tsp garlic, minced

Directions:

In a saucepan, add oil, garlic, and onion and sauté for 3 minutes over medium heat.

Add remaining ingredients into the saucepan and bring to boil.

Reduce heat and cover and simmer for 10 minutes.

Puree the soup using a blender until smooth.

Stir well and serve warm.

Roasted Squash

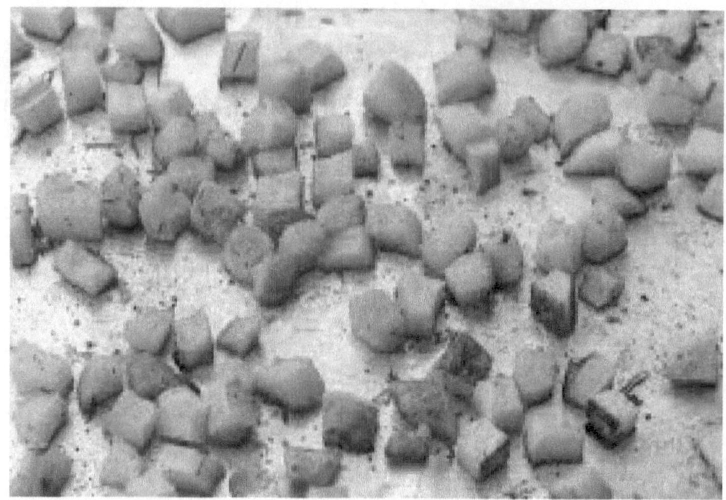

Preparation time: 1 hour 10 minutes

Servings: 3

Ingredients:

2 lbs. summer squash, cut into 1-inch pieces

1/8 tsp pepper

1/8 tsp garlic powder

3 tbsp olive oil

1 large lemon juice

1/8 tsp paprika

Pepper

Salt

Directions:

Preheat the oven to 400 F/ 204 C.

Spray a baking tray with cooking spray.

Place squash pieces onto the prepared baking tray and drizzle with olive oil.

Season with paprika, pepper, and garlic powder.

Squeeze lemon juice over the squash and bake in preheated oven for 50-60 minutes.

Serve hot and enjoy.

Lemon Garlic Mushrooms

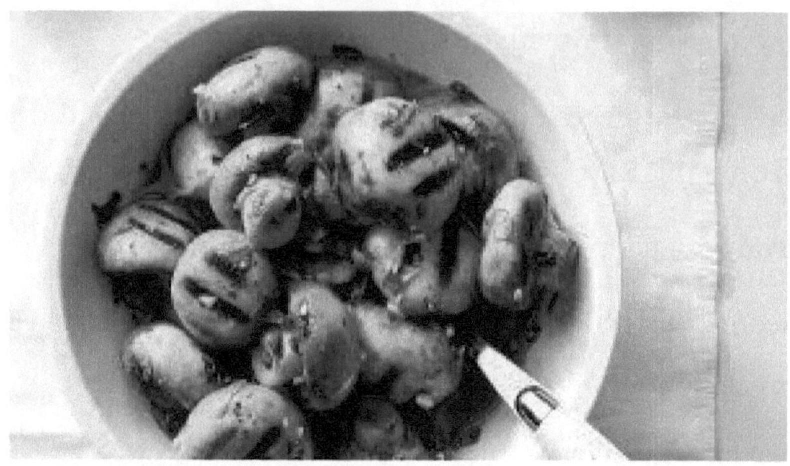

Preparation time: 25 minutes

Servings: 4

Ingredients:

3 oz enoki mushrooms

1 tbsp olive oil

1 tsp lemon zest, chopped

2 tbsp lemon juice

3 garlic cloves, sliced

6 oyster mushrooms, halved

5 oz cremini mushrooms, sliced

1/2 red chili, sliced

1/2 onion, sliced

1 tsp sea salt

Directions:

Heat olive oil in a pan over high heat.

Add shallots, enoki mushrooms, oyster mushrooms, cremini mushrooms, and chili.

Stir well and cook over medium-high heat for 10 minutes.

Add lemon zest and stir well. Season with lemon juice and salt and cook for 3-4 minutes.

Serve and enjoy.

Almond Green Beans

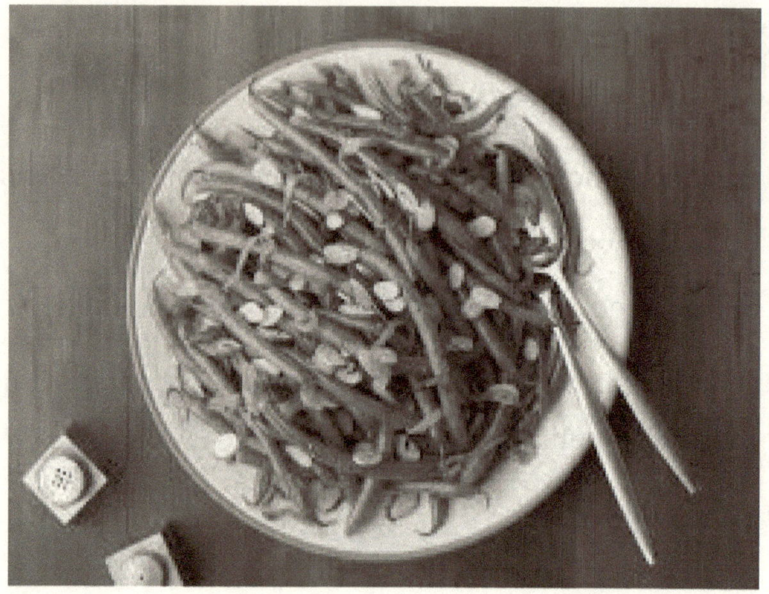

Preparation time: 20 minutes

Servings: 4

Ingredients:

1 lb fresh green beans, trimmed

1/3 cup almonds, sliced

4 garlic cloves, sliced

2 tbsp olive oil

1 tbsp lemon juice

½ tsp sea salt

Directions:

Add green beans, salt, and lemon juice in a mixing bowl. Toss well and set aside.

Heat oil in a pan over medium heat.

Add sliced almonds and sauté until lightly browned.

Add garlic and sauté for 30 seconds.

Pour almond mixture over green beans and toss well.

Stir well and serve immediately.

Fried Okra

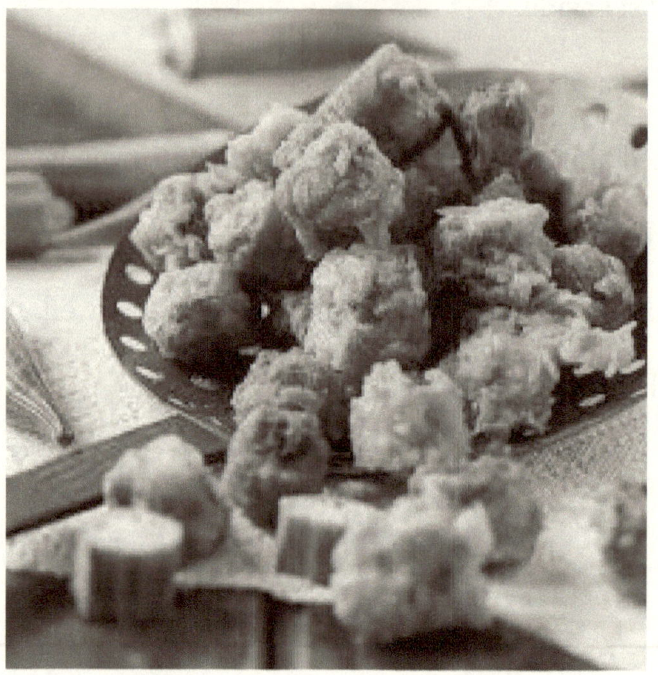

Preparation time: 20 minutes

Servings: 4

Ingredients:

1 lb fresh okra, cut into ¼" slices

1/3 cup almond meal

Pepper

Salt

Oil for frying

Directions:

Heat oil in large pan over medium-high heat.

In a bowl, mix together sliced okra, almond meal, pepper, and salt until well coated.

Once the oil is hot then add okra to the hot oil and cook until lightly browned.

Remove fried okra from pan and allow to drain on paper towels.

Serve and enjoy.

Tomato Avocado Cucumber Salad

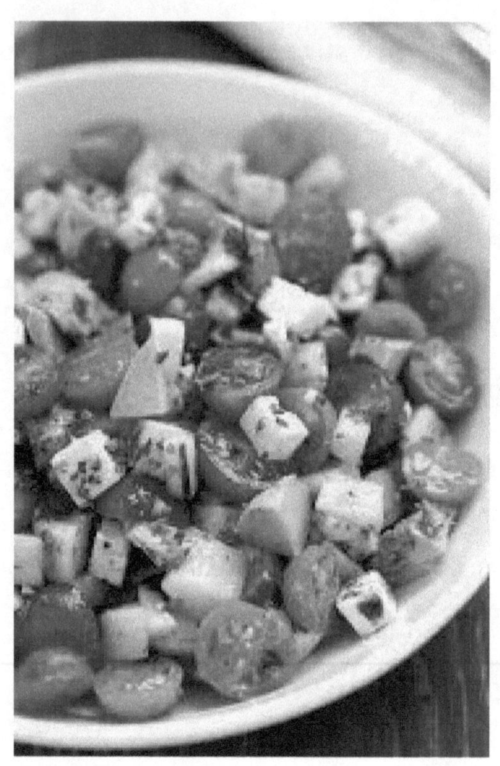

Preparation time: 10 minutes

Servings: 4

Ingredients:

1 cucumber, sliced

2 avocado, chopped

½ onion, sliced

2 tomatoes, chopped

1 bell pepper, chopped

For dressing:

2 tbsp cilantro

¼ tsp garlic powder

2 tbsp olive oil

1 tbsp lemon juice

½ tsp black pepper

½ tsp salt

Directions:

In a small bowl, mix together all dressing ingredients and set aside.

Add all salad ingredients into the large mixing bowl and mix well.

Pour dressing over salad and toss well.

Serve immediately and enjoy.

Asian Cucumber Salad

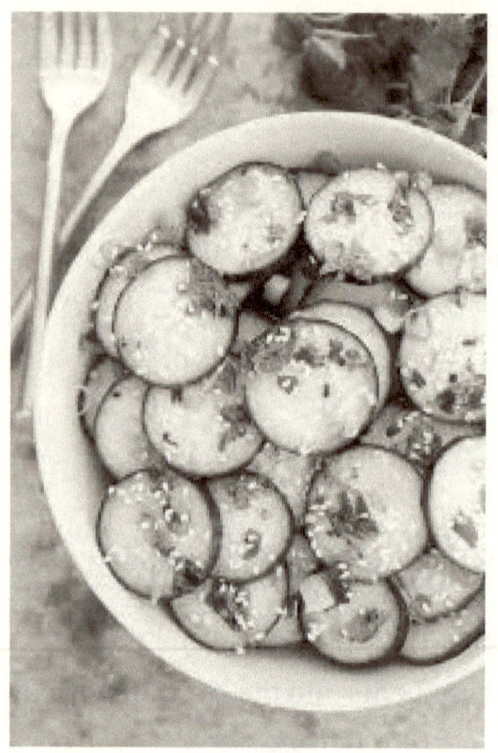

Preparation time: 10 minutes

Servings: 6

Ingredients:

4 cups cucumbers, sliced

¼ tsp red pepper flakes

½ tsp sesame oil

1 tsp sesame seeds

¼ cup rice wine vinegar

¼ cup red pepper, diced

¼ cup onion, sliced

½ tsp sea salt

Directions:

Add all ingredients into the mixing bowl and toss well.

Serve immediately and enjoy.

Chapter 7: Dinner

Truffle Parmesan Salad

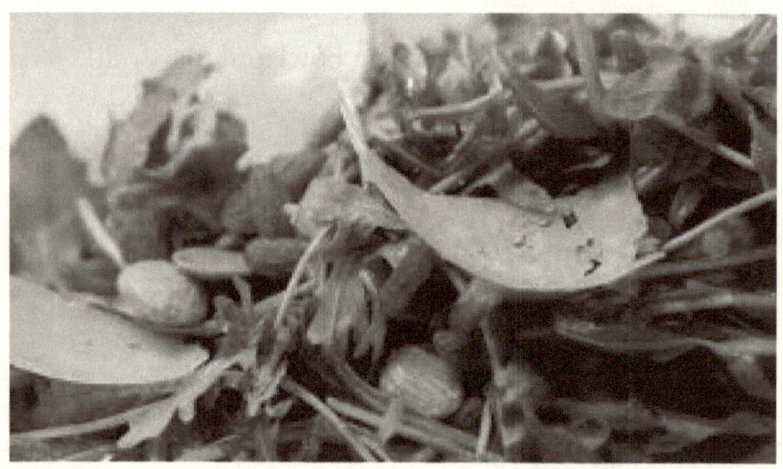

Preparation time: 15 minutes

Cooking time: 0 minutes

Servings: 4

Ingredients:

4 cups kale, chopped

½ cup truffle parmesan cheese

1 tsp. Dijon mustard

2 tbsp. olive oil

2 tbsp. lemon juice

Salt and pepper to taste

2 tbsp. water

Direction

Rinse the kale with cold water, then drain the kale and put it into a large bowl.

In a medium-sized bowl, mix the remaining ingredients into a dressing.

Pour the dressing over the kale and stir gently to cover the kale evenly.

Transfer the large bowl to the fridge and allow the salad to chill for up to one hour – doing so will guarantee a better flavor. Alternatively, the salad can be served right away. Enjoy!

Cashew Siam Salad

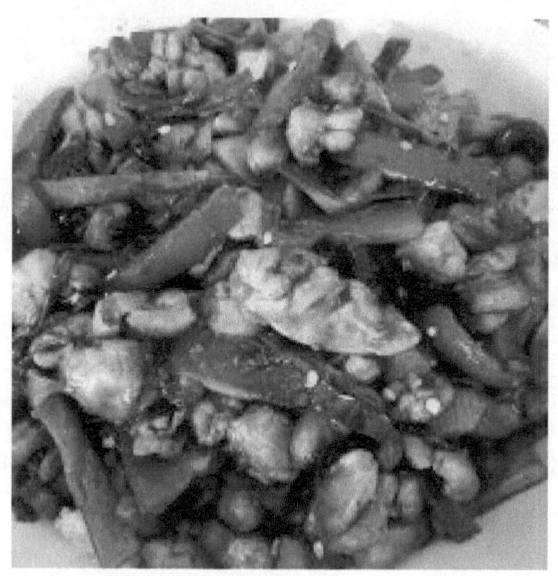

Preparation time: 12 minutes

Cooking time: 3 minutes

Servings: 4

Ingredients: Salad:

4 cups baby spinach, rinsed, drained

½ cup pickled red cabbage

Dressing:

1-inch piece ginger, finely chopped

1 tsp. chili garlic paste

1 tbsp. soy sauce

½ tbsp. rice vinegar

1 tbsp. sesame oil

3 tbsp. avocado oil

Toppings:

½ cup raw cashews, unsalted

¼ cup fresh cilantro, chopped

Direction

Put the spinach and red cabbage in a large bowl. Toss to combine and set the salad aside.

Toast the cashews in a frying pan over medium-high heat, stirring occasionally until the cashews are golden brown. This should take about 3 minutes. Turn off the heat and set the frying pan aside.

Mix all the dressing ingredients in medium-sized bowl and use a spoon to mix them into a smooth dressing.

Pour the dressing over the spinach salad and top with the toasted cashews.

Toss the salad to combine all ingredients and transfer the large bowl to the fridge. Allow the salad to chill for up to one hour – doing so will guarantee a better flavor. Alternatively, the salad can be served right away, topped with the optional cilantro. Enjoy!

Avocado and Cauliflower Hummus

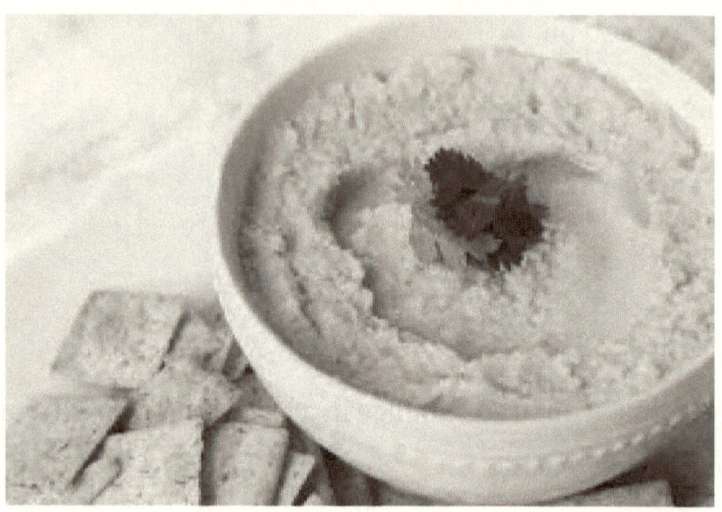

Preparation time: 5 minutes

Cooking time: 20 minutes

Servings: 2

Ingredients:

1 medium cauliflower, stem removed and chopped

1 large Hass avocado, peeled, pitted, and chopped

¼ cup extra virgin olive oil

2 garlic cloves

½ tbsp. lemon juice

½ tsp. onion powder

Sea salt and ground black pepper to taste

2 large carrots

¼ cup fresh cilantro, chopped

Direction

Preheat the oven to 450°F, and line a baking tray with aluminum foil.

Put the chopped cauliflower on the baking tray and drizzle with 2 tablespoons of olive oil.

Roast the chopped cauliflower in the oven for 20-25 minutes, until lightly brown.

Remove the tray from the oven and allow the cauliflower to cool down.

Add all the ingredients—except the carrots and optional fresh cilantro—to a food processor or blender, and blend the ingredients into a smooth hummus.

Transfer the hummus to a medium-sized bowl, cover, and put it in the fridge for at least 30 minutes.

Take the hummus out of the fridge and, if desired, top it with the optional chopped cilantro and more salt and pepper to taste; serve with the carrot fries, and enjoy!

Raw Zoodles with Avocado 'N Nuts

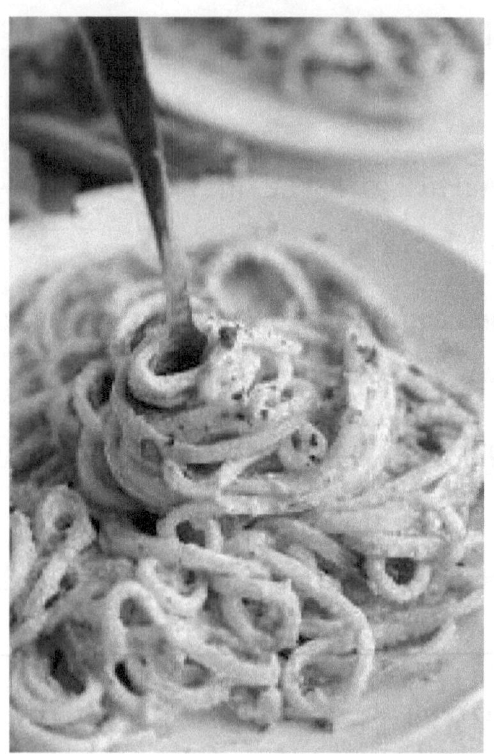

Preparation time: 10 minutes

Cooking time: 0 minutes

Servings: 2

Ingredients:

1 medium zucchini

1½ cups basil

⅓ cup water

5 tbsp. pine nuts

2 tbsp. lemon juice

1 medium avocado, peeled, pitted, and sliced

2 tbsp. olive oil

6 yellow cherry tomatoes, halved

6 red cherry tomatoes, halved

Sea salt and black pepper to taste

Direction

Add the basil, water, nuts, lemon juice, avocado slices, optional olive oil (if desired), salt, and pepper to a blender.

Blend the ingredients into a smooth mixture. Add more salt and pepper to taste and blend again.

Divide the sauce and the zucchini noodles between two medium-sized bowls for serving, and combine in each.

Top the mixtures with the halved yellow cherry tomatoes, and the optional red cherry tomatoes (if desired); serve and enjoy!

Cauliflower Sushi

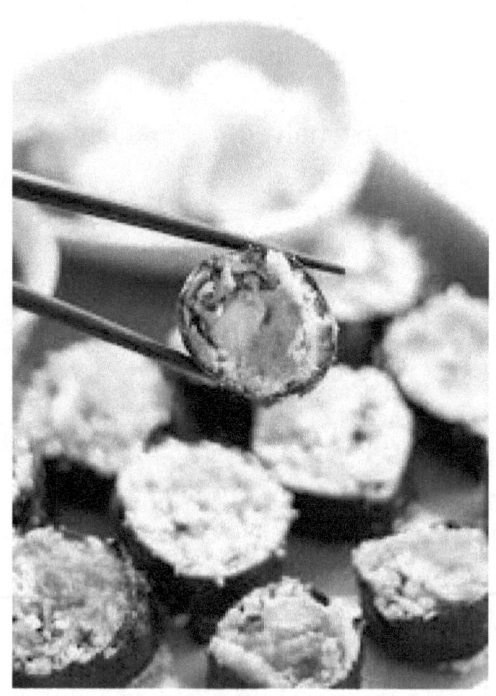

Preparation time: 30 minutes

Cooking time: 0 minutes

Servings: 4

Ingredients: Sushi Base:

6 cups cauliflower florets

½ cup vegan cheese

1 medium spring onion, diced

4 nori sheets

Sea salt and pepper to taste

1 tbsp. rice vinegar or sushi vinegar

1 medium garlic clove, minced

Filling:

1 medium Hass avocado, peeled, sliced

½ medium cucumber, skinned, sliced

4 asparagus spears

handful of enoki mushrooms

Direction

Put the cauliflower florets in a food processor or blender. Pulse the florets into a rice-like substance. When using readymade cauliflower rice, add this to the blender.

Add the vegan cheese, spring onions, and vinegar to the food processor or blender. Top these ingredients with salt and pepper to taste, and pulse everything into a chunky mixture. Make sure not to turn the ingredients into a puree by pulsing too long.

Taste and add more vinegar, salt, or pepper to taste. Add the optional minced garlic clove to the blender and pulse again for a few seconds.

Lay out the nori sheets and spread the cauliflower rice mixture out evenly between the sheets. Make sure to leave at least 2 inches of the top and bottom edges empty.

Place one or more combinations of multiple filling ingredients along the center of the spread out rice mixture. Experiment with different ingredients per nori sheet for the best flavor.

Roll up each nori sheet tightly. (Using a sushi mat will make this easier.)

Either serve the sushi as a nori roll, or, slice each roll up into sushi pieces.

Serve right away with a small amount of wasabi, pickled ginger, and soy sauce!

Spinach and Mashed Tofu Salad

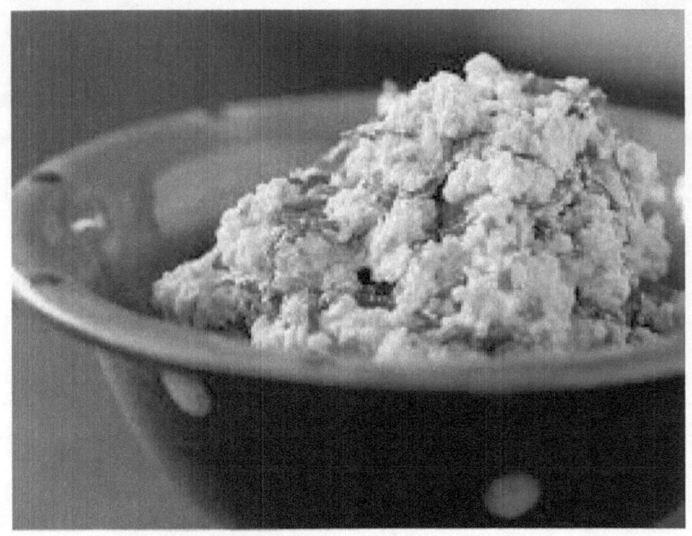

Preparation time: 20 minutes

Servings: 4

Ingredients:

2 8-oz. blocks firm tofu, drained

4 cups baby spinach leaves

4 tbsp. cashew butter

1½ tbsp. soy sauce

1-inch piece ginger, finely chopped

1 tsp. red miso paste

2 tbsp. sesame seeds

1 tsp. organic orange zest

1 tsp. nori flakes

2 tbsp. water

Direction

Use paper towels to absorb any excess water left in the tofu before crumbling both blocks into small pieces.

In a large bowl, combine the mashed tofu with the spinach leaves.

Mix the remaining ingredients in another small bowl and, if desired, add the optional water for a smoother dressing.

Pour this dressing over the mashed tofu and spinach leaves.

Transfer the bowl to the fridge and allow the salad to chill for up to one hour. Doing so will guarantee a better flavor. Or, the salad can be served right away. Enjoy!

Keto Curry Almond Bread

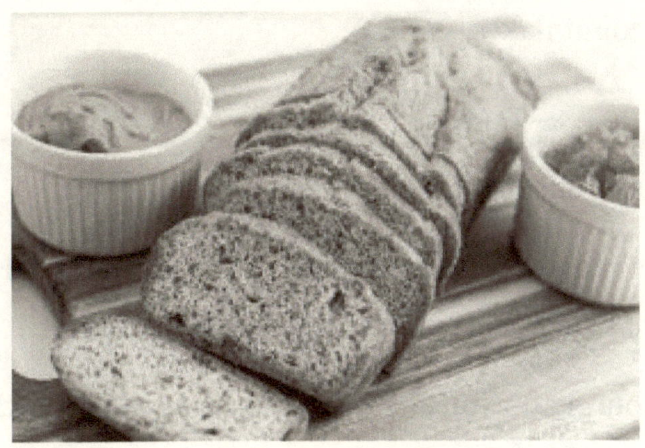

Preparation time: 10 minutes

Cooking time: 15 minutes

Servings: 2

Ingredients:

½ cup almond flour

¼ cup almond milk

¼ cup ground flaxseed

2 tbsp. coconut oil

2 tbsp. red curry paste

½ tsp. salt

½ tsp. cane sugar

2 kaffir lime leaves, chopped

2 tsp. dried ginger, fresh, minced

¼ cup water

4 tbsp. coconut flakes

Direction

Line a baking sheet with parchment paper.

In a medium bowl, mix the almond milk with the sugar, salt, and ground flaxseeds. Stir well and let it sit for 10 minutes.

Add the flour, kaffir lime leaves, and ginger to the bowl.

Incorporate all ingredients using your hands or an electric mixer. Add some of the optional water to make the mixing easier.

Divide the dough into two pieces and flatten these out onto the baking sheet.

Grease both sides of the dough with the coconut oil and apply a tablespoon of red curry paste on the top side of each flattened bread.

Allow the pieces of bread to rest for an hour at room temperature.

Preheat the oven to 400°F.

Bake the bread for about 15 minutes, until golden brown on top.

Top the breads with the optional coconut flakes.

Serve and enjoy!

Egg Roll Bowl

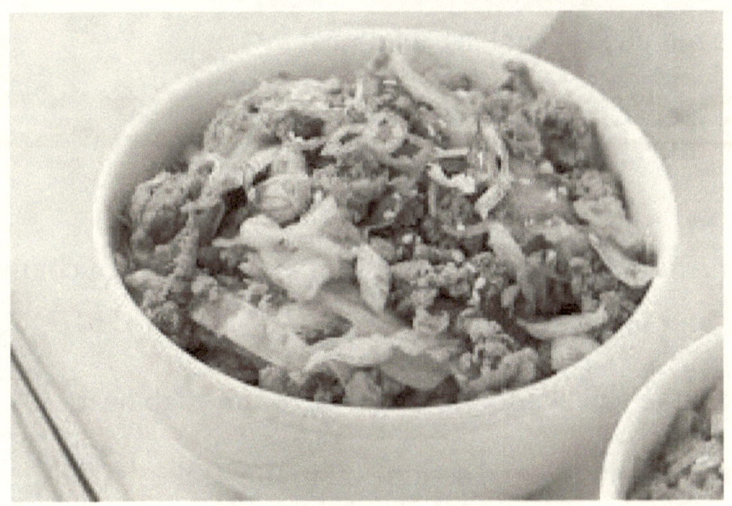

Preparation time: 5 minutes

Cooking time: 6 minutes

Servings: 2

Ingredients:

2 7-oz. packs shirataki noodles

1 tbsp. coconut oil

1 tbsp. sesame oil

1 tbsp. rice vinegar

1 12-oz. pack extra firm tofu, drained, cubed

1 red onion, diced

2 garlic cloves, minced

1-inch fresh ginger, finely minced

4 tbsp. low sodium soy sauce

½ cup red pickled cabbage, chopped

½ cup carrots, matchsticks or julienned

Direction

In a medium bowl, rinse the shirataki noodles with cold water, drain, and set aside.

Take a large skillet and put it over medium-high heat.

Add the coconut oil and sesame oil to the skillet.

Add the rice vinegar, tofu cubes, and onions to the skillet. Stir-fry the ingredients until the onions start to caramelize.

Blend in the garlic, ginger, and soy sauce. Allow the ingredients to cook for a minute while occasionally stirring.

Add the carrots to the skillet and cook for another 5 minutes while stirring occasionally.

Take the skillet off the heat, divide the shirataki noodles over 2 medium bowls, top each portion with half of the tofu mixture and chopped cabbage, serve, and enjoy!

Zoodle Pesto Salad

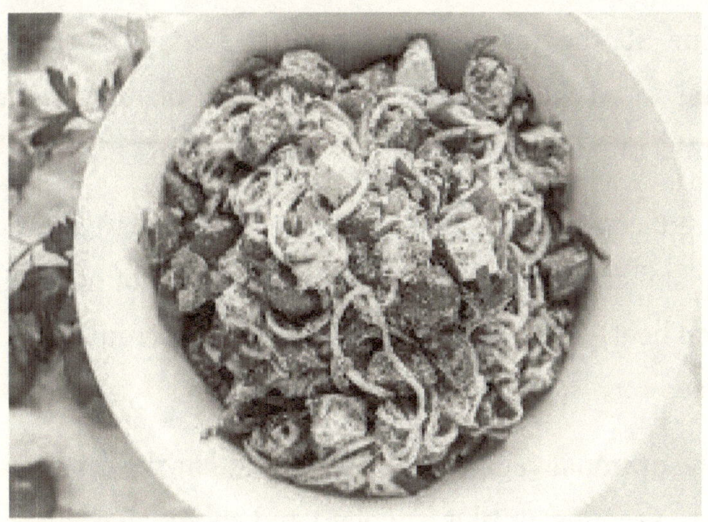

Preparation time: 20 minutes

Servings: 2

Ingredients:

2 medium zucchinis

¼ cup extra virgin olive oil

1 ½ cups fresh baby spinach leaves

¼ cup walnuts, crushed

1 tsp. garlic powder

Sea salt and ground black pepper to taste

¼ cup capers, chopped

½ cup of vegan cheese

Direction

Combine all the ingredients except the zoodles, capers, and optional vegan cheese in a food processor or blender. Pulse for 1-2 minutes into a smooth pesto.

If desired, cook zoodles or zucchini slices for up to 4 minutes in a large skillet, with boiling water and a pinch of olive oil, over medium heat. Alternatively, the zoodles or zucchini slices can be used raw.

Melt the optional vegan cheese on a plate in the microwave for about 40 seconds, until it is melted and spreadable.

Serve the raw or cooked zoodles with the pesto, garnished with the chopped capers. Top the dish with the optional molten vegan cheese and add more salt and pepper to taste.

Serve and enjoy!

Cucumber Edamame Salad

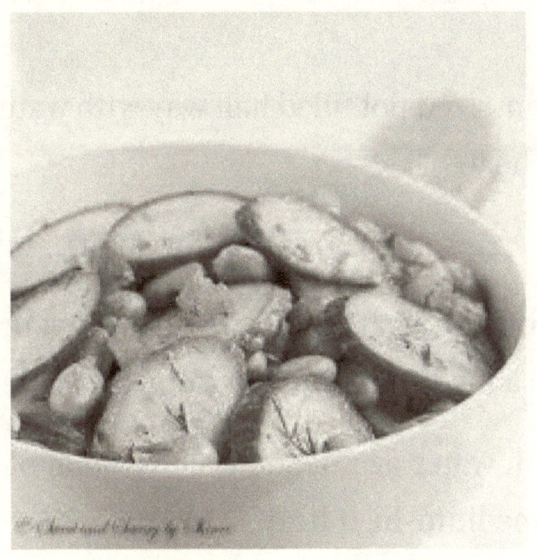

Preparation time: 5 minutes

Cooking time: 8 minutes

Servings: 2

Ingredients:

3 tbsp. avocado oil

1 cup cucumber

½ cup fresh sugar snap peas

½ cup fresh edamame

¼ cup radish, sliced

1 large Hass avocado, peeled, pitted, sliced

1 nori sheet, crumbled

2 tsp. roasted sesame seeds

1 tsp. salt

Direction

Bring a medium-sized pot filled half way with water to a boil over medium-high heat.

Add the sugar snaps and cook them for about 2 minutes.

Take the pot off the heat, drain the excess water, transfer the sugar snaps to a medium-sized bowl and set aside for now.

Fill the pot with water again, add the teaspoon of salt and bring to a boil over medium-high heat.

Add the edamame to the pot and let them cook for about 6 minutes.

Take the pot off the heat, drain the excess water, transfer the soybeans to the bowl with sugar snaps and let them cool down for about 5 minutes.

Combine all ingredients, except the nori crumbs and roasted sesame seeds, in a medium-sized bowl.

Carefully stir, using a spoon, until all ingredients are evenly coated in oil.

Top the salad with the nori crumbs and roasted sesame seeds.

Transfer the bowl to the fridge and allow the salad to cool for at least 30 minutes.

Serve chilled and enjoy!

Flourless Bread

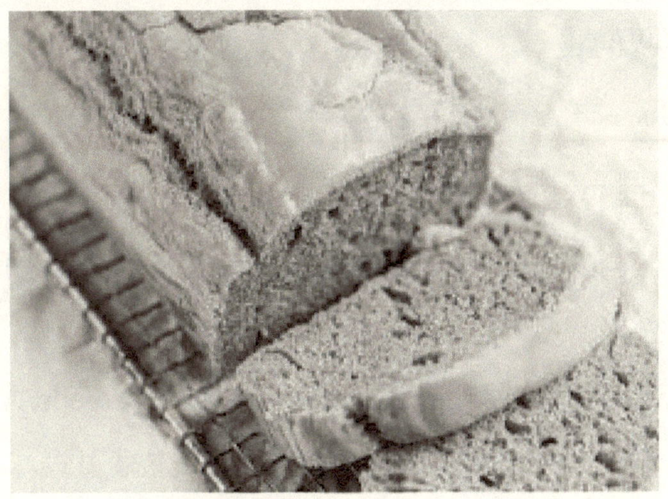

Preparation time: 5 minutes

Cooking time: 35 minutes

Servings: 12

Ingredients:

1 tsp. coconut oil

6 tbsp. water

2 tbsp. flax seed, ground

1 cup almond butter

1 cup pumpkin

1 ½ tsp. baking powder

½ tsp. cinnamon

1 cup organic soy protein, vanilla flavor

¼ cup pumpkin seeds, raw or roasted

½ tsp. nutmeg

Direction

Preheat the oven to 320°F.

Line a large loaf pan with parchment paper and grease the paper with the coconut oil.

In a small bowl, combine the water with the flax seeds. Allow the seeds to soak for about 10 minutes.

After 10 minutes, put all the ingredients except the roasted pumpkin seeds in a blender or food processor. If desired, include the optional nutmeg. Pulse until ingredients are combined into a smooth batter, scraping the sides of the blender or food processor if necessary.

Transfer the batter into the loaf pan and allow the mixture to sit for a few minutes.

Put the loaf pan in the oven and bake the bread for 20 minutes. Remove the bread and top it with the pumpkin seeds, then bake for another 15-20 minutes, or until a knife comes out clean. Take the loaf pan out of the oven and allow the bread to cool.

Transfer the bread to a cutting board and slice it into 12 slices.

Serve warm or cold and enjoy!

Walnut & Mushroom Loaf

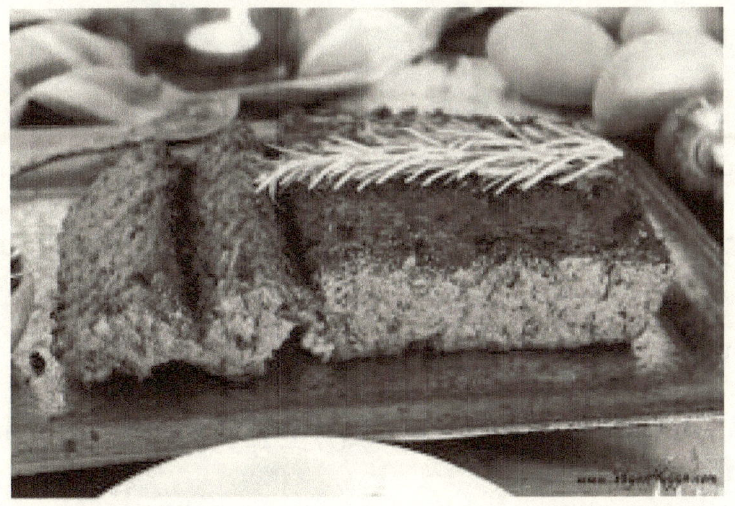

Preparation time: 5 hours

Servings: 10

Ingredients:

2 tbsp. coconut oil

2 cups walnuts

3 portobello mushroom caps, stems removed

½ cup green onion, sliced

2 cups fresh baby spinach leaves

Marinade:

1 tbsp. balsamic vinegar

1 tbsp. soy sauce

1 tsp. cumin

Pinch of Himalayan salt

Direction

Grease a large cheese mold or loaf pan that fits in a dehydrator with coconut oil and set it aside.

In a medium-sized bowl, cover the walnuts with water and soak them for at least 8 hours. Rinse and drain the walnuts after soaking, and make sure no water is left.

Mix all the marinade ingredients in a small bowl until no lumps remain.

Cut the portobello mushroom caps into small pieces. Add to the marinade bowl and stir until all pieces are evenly coated. Set the mushrooms aside for 30 minutes.

After 30 minutes, put the walnuts into a food processor or blender and pulse into tiny bits. Add the marinated mushroom pieces and green onion and continue pulsing the ingredients into a smooth mixture with tiny chunks. This should take about 2 minutes.

Transfer the mixture into the cheese mold and sprinkle with some additional salt.

Cover the mold with parchment paper and place the walnut and mushroom loaf into a dehydrator. Dehydrate the loaf at 90°F for about 2 hours.

After 2 hours, flip the mold upside down and dehydrate for another 2 hours.

Take the loaf out of the mold and cut it into 10 slices or chunks.

Serve each slice with a handful of baby spinach leaves and enjoy!

Savory Coconut Pancake

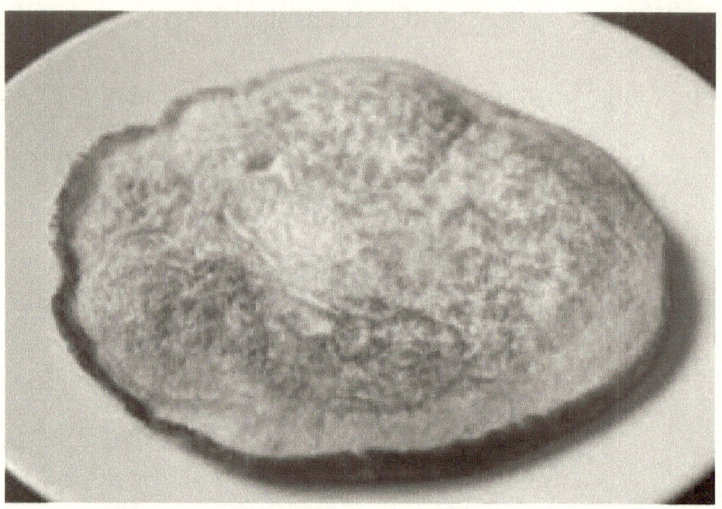

Preparation time: 12 minutes

Cooking time: 2 minutes

Servings: 1

Ingredients:

¼ cup coconut flour

¼ cup water

¼ cup green onion, diced

1 tbsp. flax seeds, ground

¼ tsp. baking powder

¼ tsp. turmeric

Sea salt and black pepper to taste

1 tsp. coconut oil

Handful fresh rocket

Direction

In a medium-sized bowl, mix all the ingredients except the coconut oil and rocket together until no lumps remain. Set the bowl aside and allow the mixture to sit for up to 5 minutes.

Put a medium-sized skillet over medium-low heat and add the coconut oil.

When the oil is shimmering, pour in the coconut flour mixture and allow the pancake to firm up.

Flip the pancake carefully by loosening the edges with a spatula, then covering the skillet with a plate, turning the skillet upside down, and sliding the pancake back into the skillet.

Cook the pancake for another 2 minutes. If desired, add seasonings to taste.

Serve the coconut pancake warm, garnished with a handful of rocket, and enjoy!

Nutritional Value Per Serving: Calories 281

Spicy Satay Tofu Salad

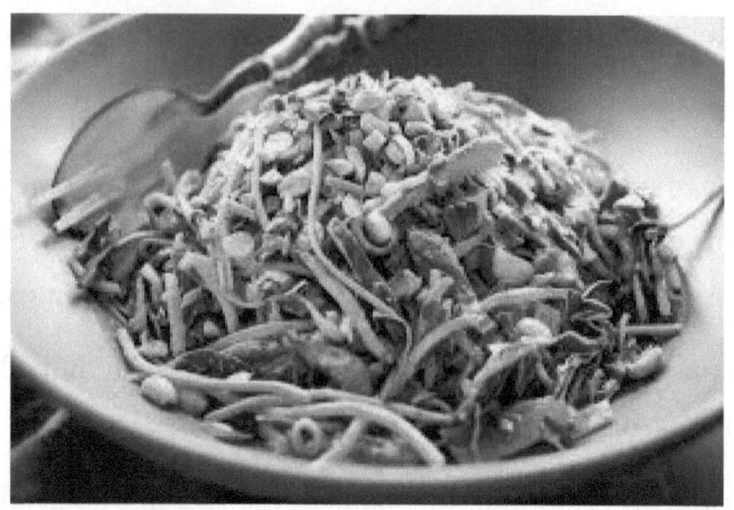

Preparation time: 8 minutes

Cooking time: 18 minutes

Servings: 2

Ingredients:

1 (12 oz. pack) extra firm tofu, drained and cubed

¼ cup peanut butter

½ tbsp. smoked paprika

1 tbsp. sesame oil

¼ tbsp. red chili flakes

2 drops liquid smoke

2 tbsp. water

1 tbsp. black sesame seeds

Salad:

4 cups fresh baby spinach leaves, rinsed, drained

¼ cup fresh mint leaves, chopped

2 tbsp. lemon juice

2 tbsp. avocado oil

¼ cup roasted cashews, unsalted

Direction

Preheat the oven to 400°F and line a baking tray with parchment paper.

Put the peanut butter, paprika, sesame oil, chili flakes and liquid smoke into a large bowl.

Add the water to the bowl and mix thoroughly until all the ingredients are combined.

Put the tofu cubes in the bowl with the peanut butter mixture and stir gently until all cubes are evenly covered.

Transfer the covered tofu cubes onto the baking tray, spread them out evenly, and sprinkle the sesame seeds over them.

Put the baking tray in the oven and bake the tofu cubes for 18 minutes, or until browned and firm.

Mix all the salad ingredients together in a large bowl.

Take the tofu out of the oven and let the cubes cool for about 2 minutes.

Divide the salad between two bowls, serve the tofu on top and enjoy!

Lemon Rosemary Almond Slices

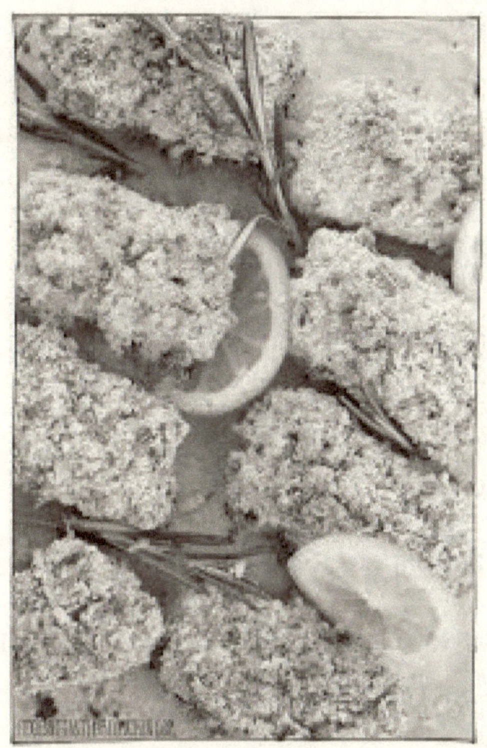

Preparation time: 5 minutes

Cooking time: 20 minutes

Servings: 4

Ingredients:

12 oz. can tofu, drained

1 cup full-fat coconut milk

1 cup almond flour

Crust:

½ cup raw almonds

1 sprig rosemary leaves, stems removed

1 tbsp. organic lemon zest

1 tsp. Himalayan salt

1 minced clove garlic

1 tsp. ground black pepper

Direction

Preheat the oven to 400°F

Line a parchment paper on baking tray.

To remove excess water on the tofu, press it on a platter and cut it into 8 slices. Set the slices aside.

Put the almonds and rosemary into a food processor and process until chunky.

Add the remaining crust ingredients to the food processor and pulse until thoroughly combined.

Transfer mixture to a bowl. Pour the coconut milk into a different medium bowl and put the almond flour in a third medium-sized bowl.

Get a tofu slice, dip every side in the almond flour. To remove excess flour shake it off.

Dip the tofu into the coconut, and then, immerse it into crust mix.

Put the tofu onto a baking tray and repeat the process for all the tofu slices. Ensure that you space the tofu slices.

Put the tray in the oven and bake for about 20 minutes, until crispy and brown.

Take the baking tray out of the oven and let the slices cool down for about a minute.

Serve alongside greens salad as a side dish and enjoy!

Stuffed Zucchini

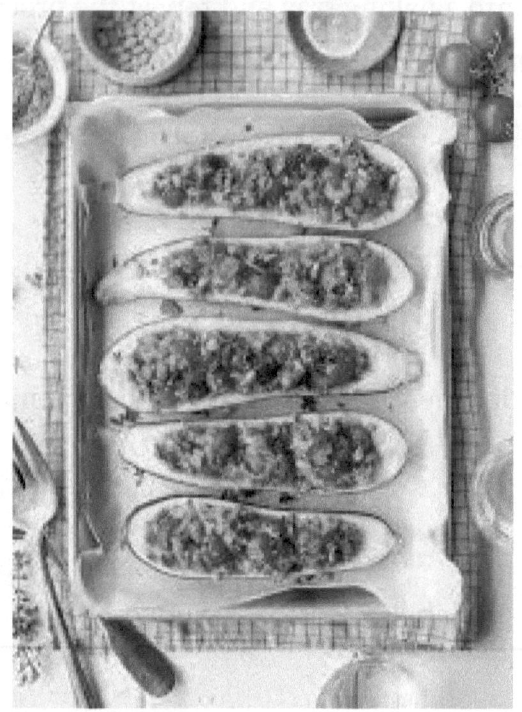

Preparation time: 5 minutes

Cooking time: 30 minutes

Servings: 2

Ingredients:

1 large zucchini

2 tbsp. olive oil

¼ cup green onion, chopped

1 garlic clove, minced

1 cup fresh baby spinach leaves

Handful of fresh rocket, chopped

Sea salt and black pepper to taste

¼ cup vegan cheese

Pinch of dried parsley

Direction

Preheat the oven to 375°F and line a baking tray with parchment paper.

Cut the zucchini in half lengthwise and scoop out most of the pulp.

Mash the zucchini pulp in a small bowl with a masher and set it aside.

Heat a large skillet over medium heat and add half of the olive oil.

Add the zucchini pulp, chopped onion, and minced garlic to the skillet.

Stir continuously, cooking the ingredients for up to 5 minutes before adding the baby spinach and rocket.

Stir for a few seconds, season with salt and pepper to taste, and turn off the heat.

Add the vegan cheese and stir well to ensure all ingredients are incorporated and the cheese has melted.

Scoop the mixture into the zucchini halves and transfer them onto the baking tray.

Cover the baking tray with aluminum foil and transfer it to the oven.

Bake the stuffed zucchini halves for 25 minutes. Then, turn off the oven, uncover the baking tray, and put the uncovered zucchini halves back into the oven for a few more minutes.

Serve the stuffed zucchini garnished with the remaining olive oil and some dried parsley.

Serve and enjoy!

Avocado Fries

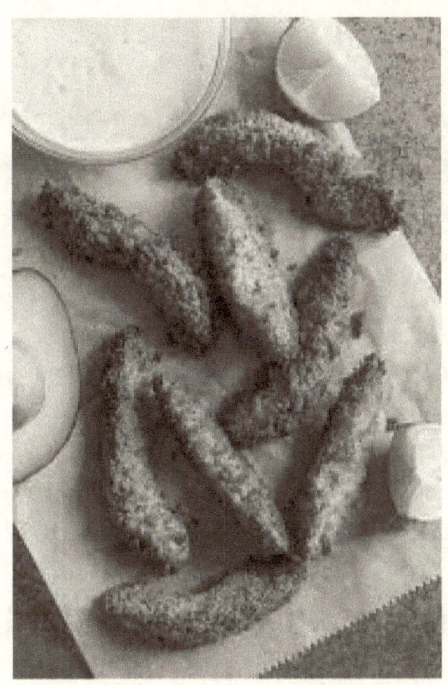

Preparation time: 3 minutes

Cooking time: 25 minutes

Servings: 2

Ingredients:

1 tbsp. olive oil

½ cup almond flour

¼ tsp. cayenne pepper

¼ tsp. smoked paprika

Pinch of salt

¾ tbsp. unsweetened almond milk

1 medium Hass avocado, pitted, peeled

1 tsp. lime juice

Direction

Preheat the oven to 400°F.

Line a baking tray with parchment paper and grease the paper with the olive oil.

In a small bowl, combine the flour, cayenne pepper, smoked paprika, and salt.

Pour the almond milk into another small bowl.

Slice the peeled avocado into 10 equally-sized fries.

Coat all sides of the fries in the flour mixture, dip in almond milk, and coat with another layer of flour.

Transfer the coated fries to the greased baking tray.

Bake the fries for 5 minutes, then flip them over and bake for another 10 minutes. Flip the fries again and bake for 5 more minutes.

Flip the fries one more time, sprinkle them with the lime juice, and bake them for a final 5 minutes.

Take the baking tray out of the oven and allow the fries to cool down for a few minutes.

Serve warm with any low-carb (vegan) sauce and enjoy!

Mushroom Zoodle Pasta

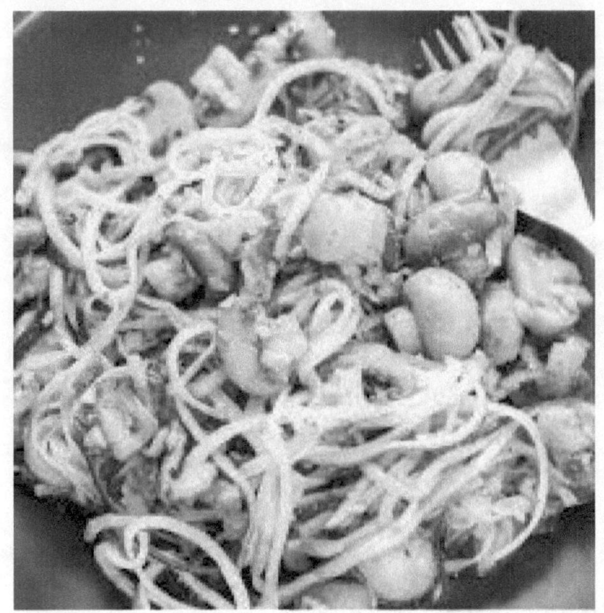

Preparation time: 10 minutes

Cooking time: 16 minutes

Servings: 4

Ingredients:

3 large zucchinis

½ tsp. salt

1 tbsp. coconut oil

1 large green onion, diced

3 garlic cloves, minced

5 cups oyster mushrooms, chopped

Pinch each of nutmeg, onion powder, paprika powder, white pepper, and salt

1 cup full-fat coconut milk

½ cup vegan mozzarella

½ cup baby spinach leaves, chopped

¼ cup fresh thyme, chopped

1 tbsp. miso paste

Direction

In a large bowl, toss the zoodles or zucchini slices with half a teaspoon of salt and set aside.

Put a large skillet, over medium heat and add the coconut oil.

Add the onion and cook until translucent, for about 5 minutes while stirring occasionally.

Stir in the minced garlic, chopped mushrooms, and remaining seasonings.

Cook all ingredients in the skillet for about 3 minutes, stirring continuously.

Reduce heat to medium-low and slowly incorporate the coconut milk, followed by the mozzarella.

Cover the skillet and let the ingredients heat through for about 8 minutes, stirring occasionally.

Drain any excess liquid from the salted zoodles by dabbing them with paper towels.

Add the dry zoodles to the skillet with the chopped spinach and stir well until all ingredients are combined.

Turn off the heat and top the mushroom zoodle pasta with the chopped thyme.

Add more seasonings to taste, serve the pasta in a bowl, and enjoy!

Quick Veggie Protein Bowl

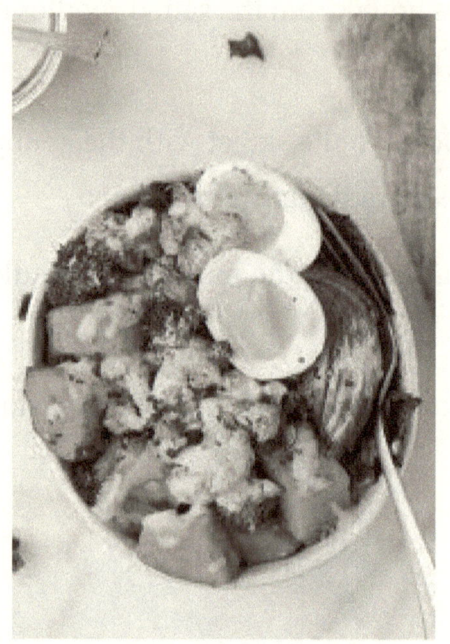

Preparation time: 5 minutes

Cooking time: 13 minutes

Servings: 1

Ingredients:

4 oz. extra-firm tofu, drained

¼ tsp. turmeric

¼ tsp. cayenne pepper

1 tbsp. coconut oil

1 cup broccoli florets, diced

1 cup Chinese kale, diced

½ cup button mushrooms, diced

½ tsp. dried oregano

Himalayan salt and ground black pepper to taste

½ tsp. paprika

¼ cup of fresh oregano, diced

Direction

Cut the tofu into tiny pieces and season with the turmeric and cayenne pepper.

Warm a large skillet over medium heat and add ¾ of the coconut oil.

Once oil is heated, add the tofu and cook it for about 5 minutes, stirring continuously.

Transfer the cooked tofu to a medium-sized bowl and set it aside.

Add the remaining coconut oil, diced broccoli florets, Chinese kale, button mushrooms, and the remaining herbs to the skillet. Season with the salt, pepper, and paprika to taste.

Cook the vegetables for 6-8 minutes, stirring continuously.

Turn off the heat and transfer the cooked veggies and tofu to the bowl. Garnish with the optional fresh oregano.

Serve and enjoy!

Cauliflower pizza crust

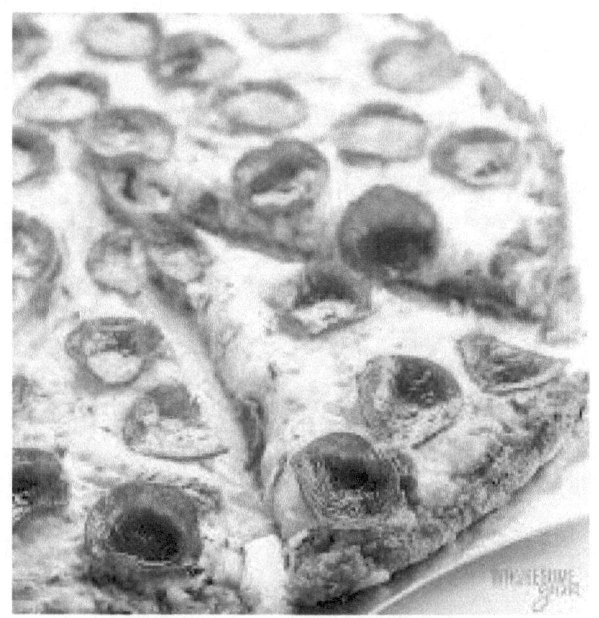

Preparation time: minutes

Cooking time: minutes

Serves:

Ingredients: Crust:

16 oz. cauliflower rice

3 flax eggs

2 tbsp. chia seeds

½ cup almond flour

½ tsp. garlic powder

½ tsp. dried basil

Pinch of salt

2 tsp. water

Topping:

½ cup simple marinara sauce

1 medium zucchini, sliced

1 medium green bell pepper, pitted, cored, sliced

1 cup button mushrooms, diced

½ cup vegan cheese

Sea salt and ground black pepper to taste

1 jalapeño pepper, pitted, cored, diced

pinch of cayenne pepper

handful of fresh rocket

Direction

Preheat the oven to 400°F and line a baking sheet with parchment paper.

Transfer the cauliflower rice to a large saucepan and add enough water to cover the 'rice.' Bring the water to a soft boil over medium heat. Cover the saucepan, turn down the heat to medium-low, and allow the rice to simmer for about 5 minutes before draining the water off. This step can be skipped if store-bought cauliflower rice is used.

Transfer the cauliflower rice onto a clean dish towel and close the cloth by holding the edges. Wring out any excess water by twisting the lower part of the towel that contains the rice.

Once the cauliflower rice is completely drained, transfer the towel to the freezer for up to 15 minutes. Doing so will cool the rice.

When the cauliflower rice has cooled completely, put it into a large bowl.

Add the flax eggs, chia seeds, almond flour, garlic, dried basil, and salt. Combine all the ingredients into a firm, kneadable dough. If the dough is too firm, add the optional 2 tablespoons of water.

Spread the dough over the entire surface of the baking dish. The uncooked crust should be about ¼-inch thick.

Bake the crust in the oven for 25 minutes, then sprinkle some additional water on top and bake for another 5 minutes. The top of the crust will turn lightly golden.

Take the baking tray out of the oven and allow the crust to cool for a few minutes.

Spread the marinara sauce evenly over the golden crust. Do the same for the vegetables.

Finally, garnish the pizza with the vegan cheese, optional jalapeño, and cayenne pepper.

Season the pizza with salt and pepper and transfer it back into the oven for a few more minutes.

Serve the pizza warm, garnished with a handful of fresh rocket, and enjoy!

Tofu Cheese Nuggets & Zucchini Fries

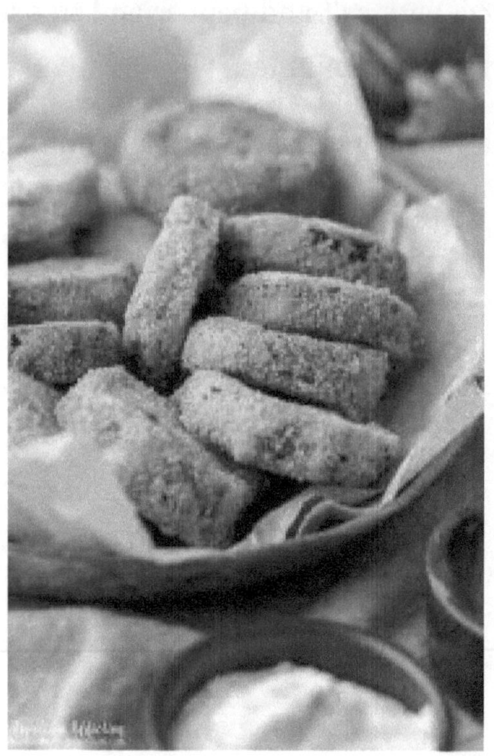

Preparation time: 5 minutes

Cooking time: 18 minutes

Servings: 2

Ingredients: Tof u Cheese Nuggets:

1 (12 oz. pack) extra firm tofu, drained, cubed

½ cup smoked chipotle cream cheese

½ cup almond flour

2 tbsp. water

Zucchini Fries:

2 tsp. red chili flakes

½ cup almond flour

¼ cup olive oil

1 large zucchini, skinned

Direction

Preheat the oven to 400°F and line a baking tray with parchment paper.

Put the cream cheese, ½ cup almond flour, and water into a large bowl and mix thoroughly until all the ingredients are combined.

Add the tofu cubes to the bowl and coat all the cubes evenly.

Transfer the coated tofu cubes onto one half of the baking tray and set it aside.

Put the chili flakes and almond flour into a large bowl and mix until all ingredients are combined.

Pour the olive oil into a medium-sized bowl and dip each zucchini stick into the oil. Make sure to cover all fries evenly.

Put the zucchini fries in the bowl with the almond flour mixture and gently stir the fries around until they are all evenly covered.

Transfer the zucchini fries onto the baking tray with the tofu nuggets and spread them out evenly. If the nuggets and fries don't fit on the baking tray together, bake them in two batches.

Put the baking tray into the oven and bake the nuggets and fries for about 18 minutes, or until golden-brown and crispy.

Take the baking tray out of the oven and let the dish cool down for about a minute.

Serve and enjoy with a light salad of greens as a side dish.

Avocado Spring Rolls

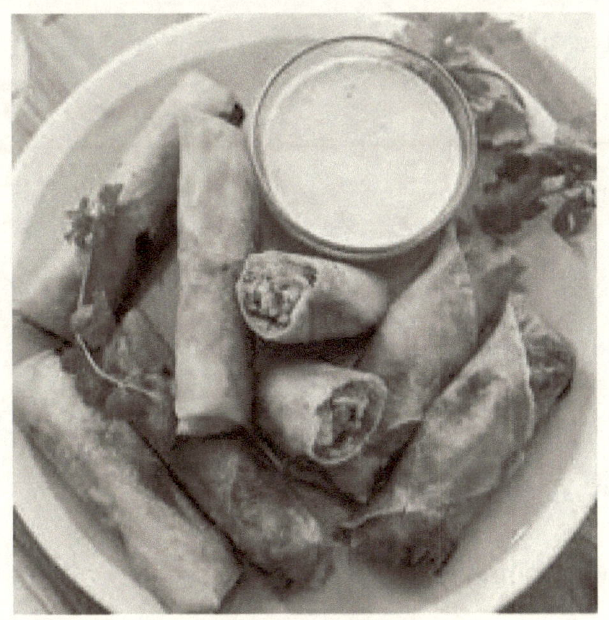

Preparation time: 20 minutes

Cooking time: 1 minutes

Servings: 4

Ingredients:

2 medium Hass avocados, peeled, pitted, sliced

1-inch piece ging er, grated

1 garlic clove, minced

Juice of ½ lemon

½ cup cabbage, shredded

¼ cup carrots, julienned or matchsticks

4-6 coconut wraps

2 tbsp. olive oil

Spicy Almond Sauce:

½ cup almond butter

2 tsp. low-sodium soy sauce

½ tsp. rice vinegar

Juice of ½ lemon

½ tsp. chili garlic paste

1 tbsp. low-carb maple syrup

2 tsp. sesame oil

Direction

In a small bowl, gently toss together the sliced avocado, ginger, garlic, lemon juice, cabbage, and julienned carrots.

Put a coconut wrap on a flat and dry surface. Place about ¼ of the avocado mixture in the center of the wrap.

Fold the wrap about ½ inch inward on two parallel sides and roll the wrap up until the mixture is covered.

Repeat with the remaining 3-5 wraps until all of the avocado mixture is used.

Put a skillet over medium-high heat and warm the olive oil until shimmering.

Add the spring rolls to the skillet and brown them, about 30 seconds on each side.

Prepare the sauce by putting all the sauce ingredients into a medium-sized bowl and stir thoroughly. Add one or more tablespoon of warm water, if necessary, to achieve the desired consistency.

Serve the spring rolls warm with the spicy almond sauce as a dip and enjoy!

Cauliflower Curry Soup

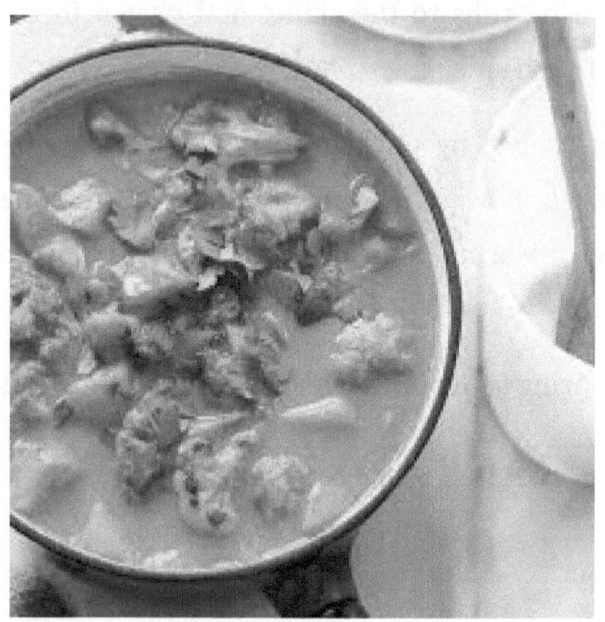

Preparation time: 5 minutes

Cooking time: 40 minutes

Servings: 4

Ingredients:

1 large cauliflower, chopped

4 tbsp. olive oil

½ red onion, finely chopped

4 garlic cloves, minced

1 tbsp. yellow curry paste

1-inch piece ginger, grated

1 (12 oz. pack) extra firm tofu, drained, scrambled

1 tsp. chili flakes

Juice of 1 medium lime

4 cups vegetable broth

1 tbsp. sesame oil

1 tsp. low-sodium soy sauce

1 cup full-fat coconut milk

Direction

Preheat the oven to 400°F and line a baking tray with parchment paper.

Put the cauliflower florets on the baking tray and drizzle 2 tablespoons of olive oil over them, covering them evenly.

Put the baking tray into the oven and bake for about 25-30 minutes, until the florets are golden brown.

Put a large pot over medium heat and add the remaining 2 tablespoons of olive oil.

Take the baking tray out of the oven and set it aside for a few minutes to let the cauliflower florets cool down.

Add the onion and garlic to the pot and fry for about a minute, stirring occasionally.

Add the curry paste to the pot along with the ginger, scrambled tofu, and chili flakes. Stir for another minute.

Put the baked cauliflower florets into a blender or food processor, along with the vegetable broth, sesame oil, soy sauce, and coconut milk.

Blend these ingredients until smooth, then transfer the mixture into the pot.

Incorporate all the ingredients, stirring occasionally until the contents of the pot start to cook. Once the soup reaches the boiling point, bring the heat down to a simmer.

Cover the pot and let the soup simmer for about 10 minutes, then take the pot off the heat and set it aside to cool for a few minutes.

Enjoy!

Roasted Vegetables with Herbs

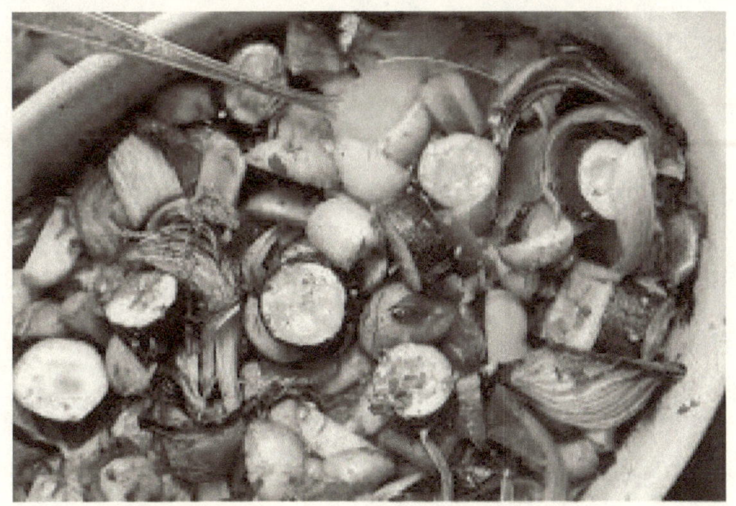

Preparation time: 10 minutes

Cooking time: 40 minutes

Servings: 4

Ingredients:

1 red bell pepper, deveined and sliced

1 green bell pepper, devein ed and sliced

1 orange bell pepper, deveined and sliced

½ head of cauliflower, broken into large florets

2 zucchinis, cut into thick slices

2 medium-sized leeks, quartered

4 garlic cloves, halved

2 thyme sprigs, chopped

1 teaspoon dried sage, crushed

4 tablespoons olive oil

4 tablespoons tomato puree

1 teaspoon mixed whole peppercorns

Sea salt and cayenne pepper, to taste

Direction

Preheat your oven to 425°F. Sprits a rimmed baking sheet with a nonstick cooking spray.

Toss all of the above vegetables with the seasonings, oil and apple cider vinegar.

Roast about 40 minutes. Flip the vegetables halfway through the cooking time. Bon appétit!

Chapter 8: Dessert and snacks

Lemon Mousse

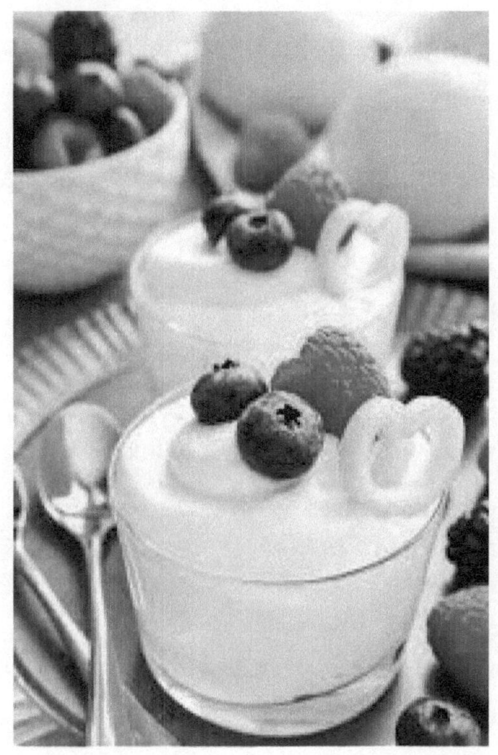

Preparation time: 10 minutes

Servings: 2

Ingredients:

14 oz coconut milk

12 drops liquid stevia

1/2 tsp lemon extract

1/4 tsp turmeric

Directions:

Place coconut milk can in the refrigerator for overnight. Scoop out thick cream into a mixing bowl.

Add remaining ingredients to the bowl and whip using a hand mixer until smooth.

Transfer mousse mixture to a zip-lock bag and pipe into small serving glasses. Place in refrigerator.

Serve chilled and enjoy.

Avocado Pudding

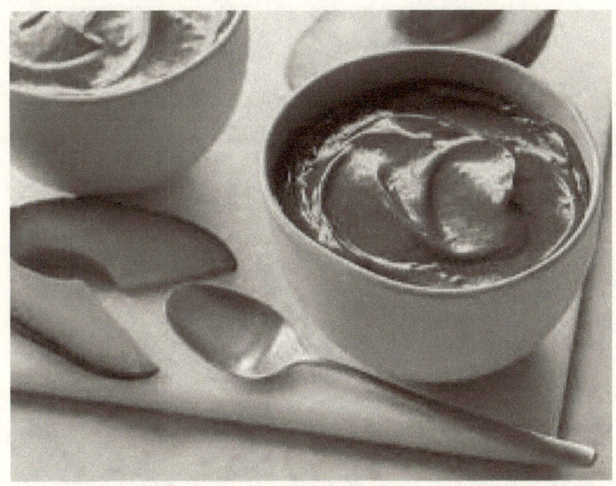

Preparation time: 10 minutes

Servings: 8

Ingredients:

2 ripe avocados, peeled, pitted and cut into pieces

1 tbsp fresh lime juice

14 oz can coconut milk

80 drops of liquid stevia

2 tsp vanilla extract

Directions:

Add all ingredients into the blender and blend until smooth.

Serve and enjoy.

Almond Butter Brownies

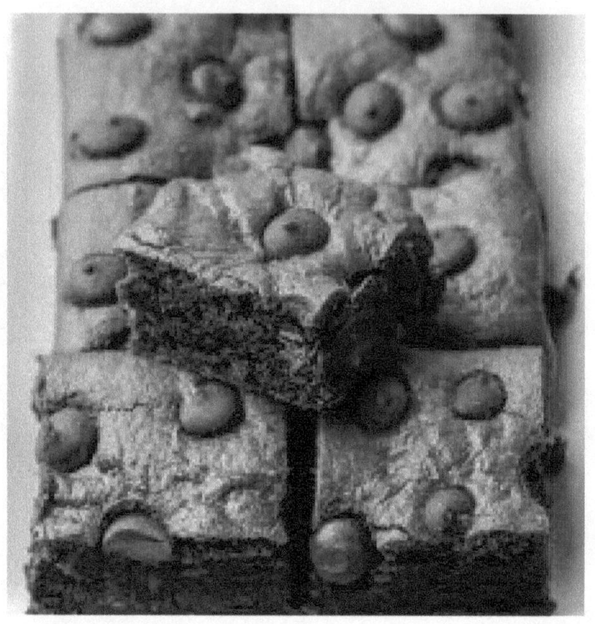

Preparation time: 30 minutes

Servings: 4

Ingredients:

1 scoop protein powder

2 tbsp cocoa powder

1/2 cup almond butter, melted

1 cup bananas, overripe

Directions:

Preheat the oven to 350 F/ 176 C.

Spray brownie tray with cooking spray.

Add all ingredients into the blender and blend until smooth.

Pour batter into the prepared dish and bake in preheated oven for 20 minutes.

Serve and enjoy.

Simple Almond Butter Fudge

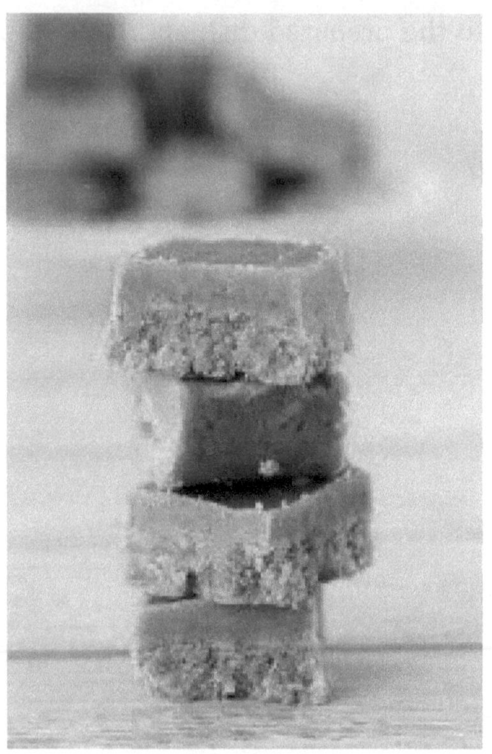

Preparation time: 15 minutes

Servings: 8

Ingredients:

1/2 cup almond butter

15 drops liquid stevia

2 1/2 tbsp coconut oil

Directions:

Combine together almond butter and coconut oil in a saucepan. Gently warm until melted.

Add stevia and stir well.

Pour mixture into the candy container and place in refrigerator until set.

Serve and enjoy.

Crispy Squash Chips

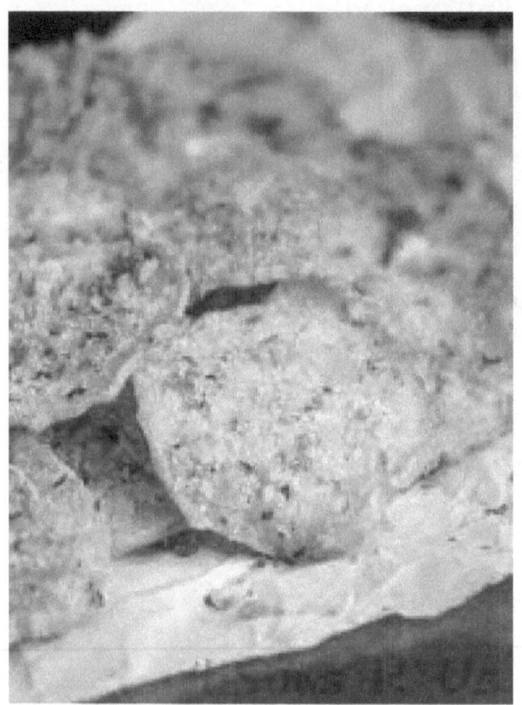

Preparation time: 30 min.

Servings: 2

Ingredients:

1 t. cayenne pepper

1 t. cumin

1 t. paprika

1 tbsp. avocado oil

1 medium butternut squash, skinny neck

Sea salt to taste

Direction:

Set the oven to 375 heat setting.

Prepare the butternut squash by removing the top.

Using a mandolin, cut the squash into even slices; it is not necessary to skin the squash.

In a big mixing bowl, place your slices of squash and cover with oil, using your hands to mix them well. Ensure all slices are oiled.

Line a cookie sheet with parchment paper and spread out your slices, so they do not overlap.

In a little bowl, mix together cayenne pepper, paprika, and cumin then sprinkle the chips over the top.

Season with sea salt to taste

Once cool, enjoy alone or with your favorite dip.

Paprika Nuts

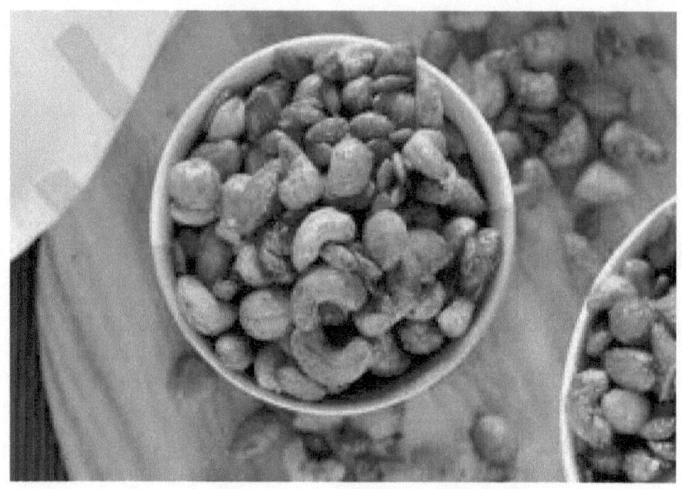

Preparation time: 30 min.

Servings: 8

Ingredients:

1 ½ t. smoked paprika

1 t. salt

2 tbsp. garlic-infused olive oil

1 c. of the following:

cashews

almonds

pecans

walnuts

Direction:

Adjust the racks in the oven so that there is one rack in the middle.

Set the oven to 325 before you start preparing the ingredients.

In a big mixing bowl, toss the nuts.

Pour olive oil over the nuts and toss to coat all the nuts.

Sprinkle the salt and paprika over the nuts and mix well. If you want more paprika flavor, then add additional paprika.

Line a big cookie sheet with parchment and spread the nuts out in one layer.

Bake for approximately 15 minutes, then remove from oven and let cool.

Enjoy.

Basil Zoodles and Olives

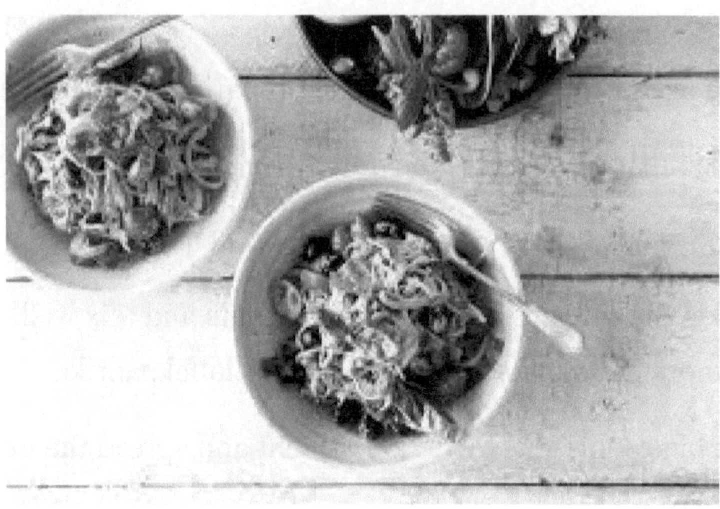

Preparation time: 4 hr. 30 min.

Servings: 6

Ingredients:

1 can black olives pitted

1 little container cherry tomatoes, halved

4 medium-size zucchini

Sauce:

½ c basil leaves, chopped

½ t. pink Himalayan salt

2 t. nutritional yeast

1 tbsp. lemon juice

½ c. water

¼ c. of the following:

sunflower seeds, soaked

cashew nuts, soaked

Direction:

Begin by preparing the sunflower seeds and cashews. Place each in a little bowl and cover with water. Allow to soak for 4 hours then drain and rinse well.

Next, place the seeds and cashews into a blender and mix until completely blended. Then add in basil, salt, nutritional yeast, lemon juice, and water. Blend until a smooth sauce is formed.

Using a spiralizer, make the zoodles from the zucchini.

Place the zoodles in a big serving bowl and then pour the sauce over the top. Stir to combine.

Top with cherry tomatoes and olives.

Serve and enjoy.

Roasted Beetroot Noodles

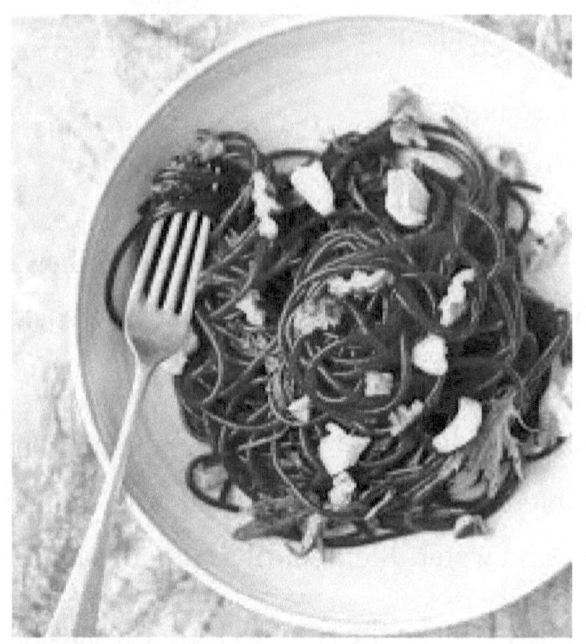

Preparation time: 35 min.

Servings: 4

Ingredients:

1 t. orange zest

2 tbsp. of the following:

parsley, chopped

balsamic vinegar

olive oil

2 big beets, peeled and spiraled

Direction:

Set the oven to 425 high-heat setting.

In a big bowl, combine the beet noodles, olive oil, and vinegar. Toss until well-combined. Season with salt and pepper to your liking.

Line a big cookie sheet with parchment paper, and spread the noodles out into a single layer. Roast the noodles for 20 minutes.

Place into bowls and zest with orange and sprinkle parsley. Gently toss and serve.

Turnip Fries

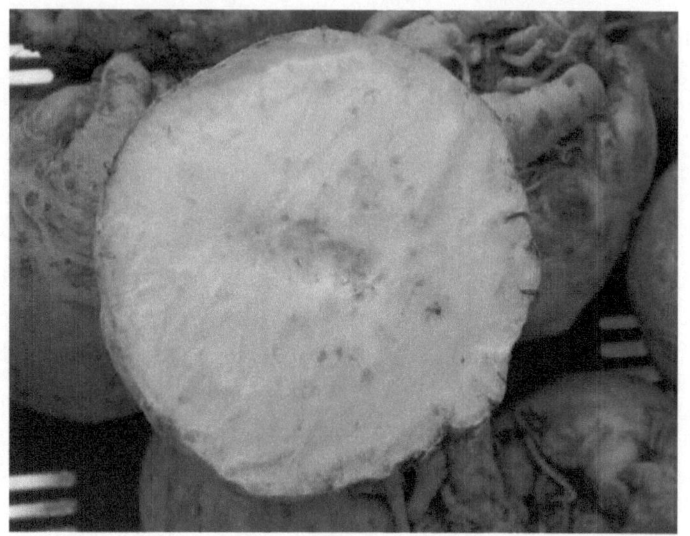

Preparation time: 45 min.

Servings: 4

Ingredients:

1 t. of the following:

onion powder

paprika

garlic salt

1 tbsp. vegetable oil

3 pounds turnips

Direction:

Set the oven to 425 heat setting.

Prepare a lightly greased aluminum foil-lined cookie sheet

Using a hand peeler, peel the turnips. With a Mandolin, cut the turnips into French fry sticks. Then place in a big bowl.

Toss the turnips with oil to coat then season with onion powder, paprika, and garlic and coat again.

Spread evenly across the cookie sheet.

Bake for 20 minutes or until the outside is crisp.

Serve with your favorite sauce or enjoy alone.

Lime and Chili Carrots Noodles

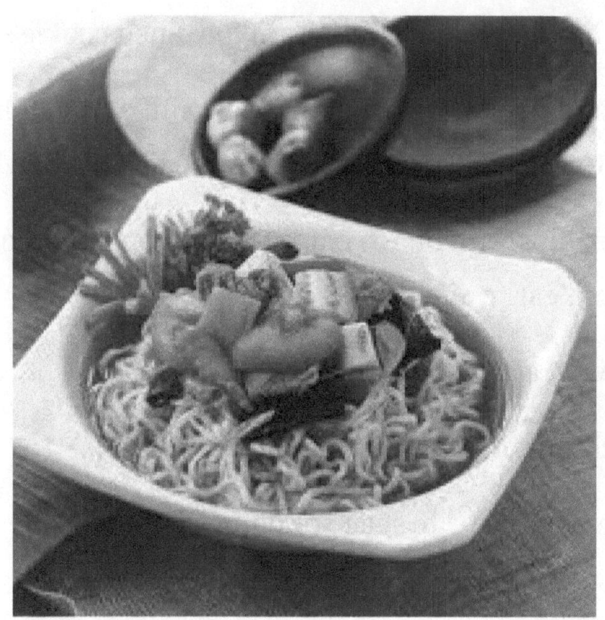

Preparation time: 10 min.

Servings: 4

Ingredients:

½ t. of the following:

black pepper

salt

2 tbsp. coconut oil

¼ c. coriander, finely chopped

2 Jalapeno chili's

1 tbsp. lime juice

2 carrots, peeled and spiralized

Direction:

In a little bowl, combine jalapeno, lime juice, and coconut oil to form a sauce.

In a big bowl, place the carrot noodles and pour dressing over the top.

Toss to ensure the dressing fully coats the noodles.

Season with salt and pepper to your liking.

Serve and enjoy.

Pesto Zucchini Noodles

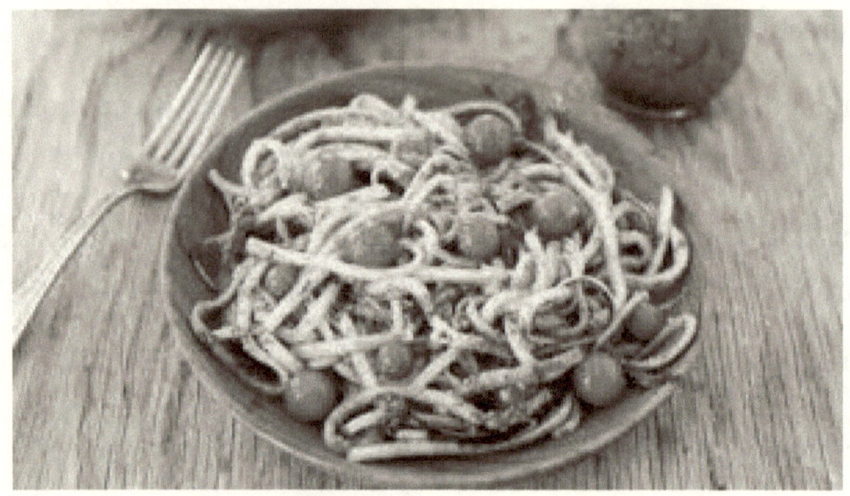

Preparation time: 15 min.

Servings:

Ingredients:

4 little zucchini ends trimmed

Cherry tomatoes

2 t. fresh lemon juice

1/3 c olive oil (best if extra-virgin)

2 cups packed basil leaves

2 c. garlic

Salt and pepper to taste

Direction:

Spiral zucchini into noodles and set to the side.

In a food processor, combine the basil and garlic and chop. Slowly add olive oil while chopping. Then pulse blend it until thoroughly mixed.

In a big bowl, place the noodles and pour pesto sauce over the top. Toss to combine.

Garnish with tomatoes and serve and enjoy.

Cabbage Slaw

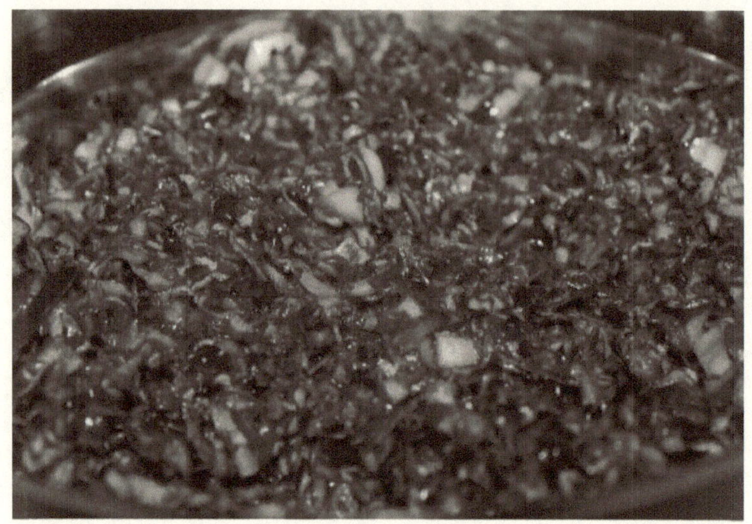

Preparation time: 5 min.

Servings: 6

Ingredients:

1/8 t. celery seed

¼ t. salt

2 tbsp. of the following:

apple cider vinegar

sweetener of your choice

½ c. vegan mayo

4 c. coleslaw mix with red cabbage and carrots

Direction:

In a big mixing bowl, whisk together the celery seed, salt, apple cider vinegar, sweetener, and vegan mayo.

Add the coleslaw and stir until appropriately combined.

Refrigerate while covered for a minimum of 2 hours or overnight if you're not in a hurry.

Garnish with tomatoes and serve and enjoy.

Zucchini Chips

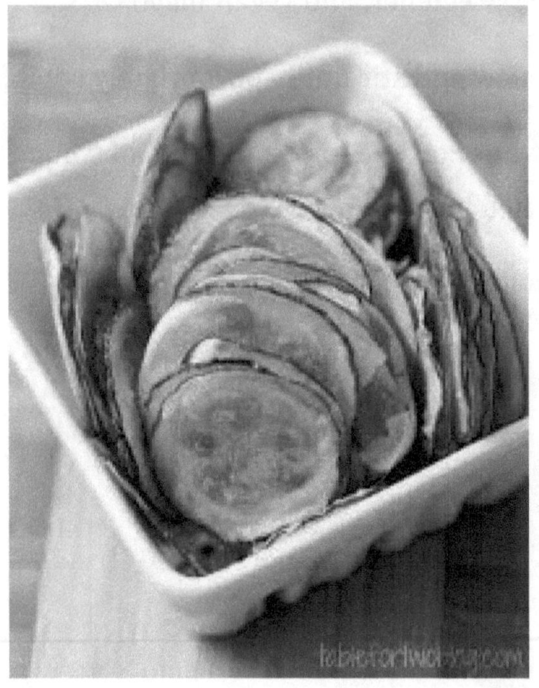

Preparation time: 1 hr. 40 min

Servings: 4

Ingredients:

2 tbsp. olive oil (best if extra virg in)

1 big zucchini

½ t. of the following:

black pepper, ground

salt

Direction:

Bring the oven to 400 heat setting.

Using a mandolin, slice the zucchini into 1/8th-inch slices.

Once sliced, use a paper towel to remove the excess moisture from the zucchini by blotting the tops.

Prepare two cookie sheets with parchment paper, and spread the zucchini out into a single layer.

Whisk well the olive oil and seasonings. With this mixture, brush each zucchini.

Bake this for 60 minutes then flip.

Check every 20 minutes, and once the zucchini is crispy, remove from the oven and serve.

Peanut Tofu Wrap

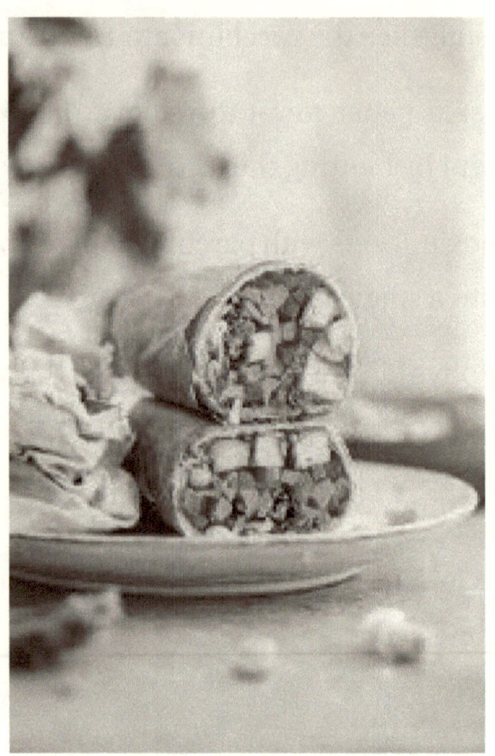

Preparation time: 30 min

Servings: 4

Ingredients:

¼ c. cilantro, finely chopped

1 c. of the following:

Asian pear

English cucumber

1 ½ t. lime zest

1 tbsp. of the following:

rice vinegar

canola oil

5 tbsp. peanut sauce

14 oz. tofu, extra firm

8 cabbage leaves

Direction:

Prepare cabbage leaves by washing and drying. Be sure to remove any stems or ribs.

Place the tofu on a paper towel-lined plate and blot to remove the extra moisture.

Set a big nonstick skillet over medium-high heat and place the oil. Once the oil is warm, add the tofu and crumble it to cook, stirring often. Wait for approximately 5 minutes or until the tofu turns golden brown. Remove from the heat and set to the side.

Mix well using a spatula the liquid ingredients, except the oil, and add the lime zest.

Add the sauce to the skillet and combine.

Place the cabbage leaves on the plates and spoon the tofu mixture into the center, topping it with cilantro, cucumber, and pear.

Cinnamon Granola

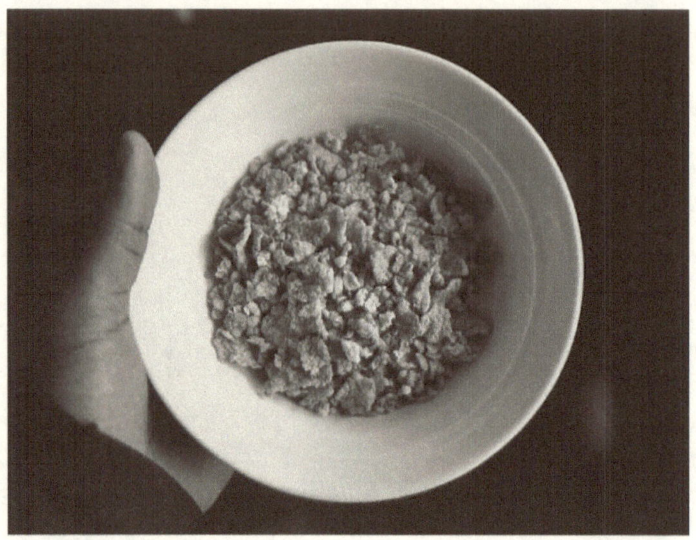

Preparation time: 25 min

Servings: 4

Ingredients:

1 ½ t. cinnamon, ground

4 tbsp. maple syrup

1/5 oz. nuts

1 tbsp. chia seeds

5 tbsp. of the following:

coconut flakes, unsweetened

flaxseed meal

Direction:

Bring the oven to 350 heat setting.

In a medium mixing bowl, combine the flaxseed, coconut, chia seed, nuts, and maple syrup. Mix well until combined.

Line a cookie sheet with parchment and spread the mixture in a single layer on the cookie sheet.

Across the top, sprinkle the cinnamon.

Place the cookie sheet in the oven, and wait for 20 minutes, approximately.

Once done, take it out and allow the granola to cool while still on the sheet.

Once cool, crumble to your desired liking and enjoy.

Chocolate Granola

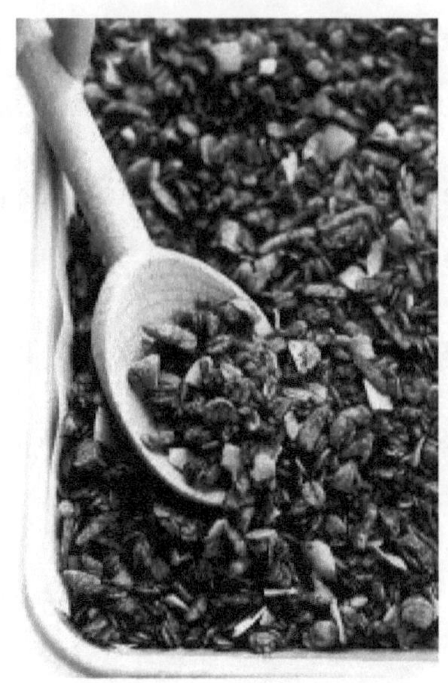

Preparation time: 60 min

Servings: 12

Ingredients:

¼ t. sea salt

¼ c. of the following:

hot water

cocoa powder

1/3 c. of the following:

coconut oil

maple syrup, sugar-free

½ c. of the following:

almond butter

almond flour

cashews, chopped

1 c. mixed seeds (flaxseed, sesame, sunflower, pumpkin)

2 c. coconut, flaked

2/3 c. almonds, flaked

Direction:

Bring the oven to 300 heat setting.

In a little bowl, mix cocoa and hot water to form a thick paste.

Next, add to the little bowl the coconut oil, maple syrup, nut butter, and salt; mix until combined thoroughly.

In a big bowl, mix the almond meal, coconut flakes, seeds, and nuts.

Transfer the chocolate mixture to the big bowl and combine well.

Using a parchment-lined cookie sheet, spread out the granola mixture.

Bake for 40 minutes or until firm.

Allow to completely cool on the parchment.

Once cool, crumble to your desired liking and enjoy.

Radish Chips

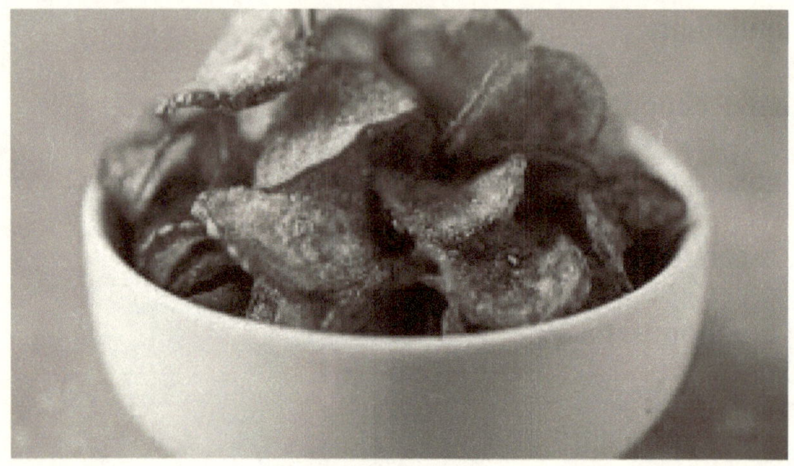

Preparation time: 1 hr. 40 min

Servings: 4

Ingredients:

2 tbsp. olive oil (best if extra virgin)

16 oz. radishes

½ t. of the following:

Black pepper, ground

Salt

Direction:

Bring the oven to 400 heat setting.

Using a mandolin, slice the radishes into 1/8**th**-inch slices.

Once sliced, use a paper towel to remove the excess moisture from the radishes by blotting the tops.

Prepare two cookie sheets with parchment paper, and spread the zucchini out into a single layer.

Add the seasonings in a bowl, with the olive oil. Whisk well and then brush each radish with this mixture, coating evenly and generously.

Bake for 10 minutes and then flip

Check every 5 minutes; once the radish is crispy, remove from the oven and serve.

Asparagus Fries

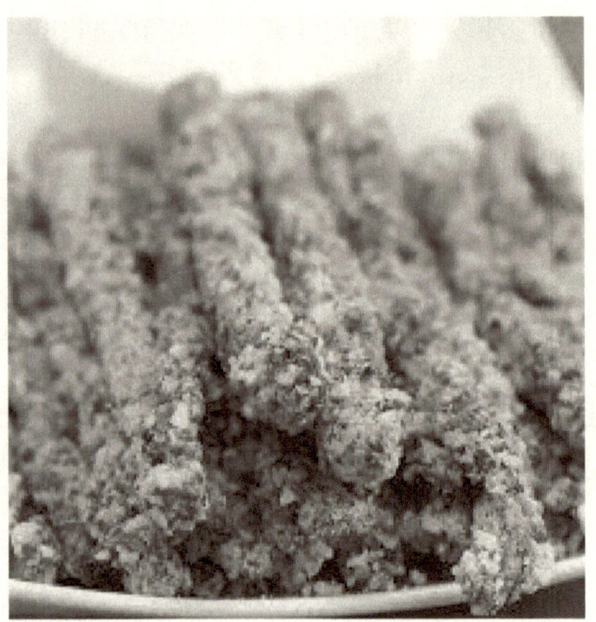

Preparation time: 1 hr. 35 min

Servings: 4

Ingredients:

2 tbsp. nutritional yeast

1 c. almond meal

1 t. of the following:

maple syrup

smoked paprika

Himalayan pink salt

½ t. black pepper, ground

1 t. extra virgin olive oil

1 bunch asparagus

Direction:

Set the oven to 400.

Prepare the asparagus by washing and cutting into equal halves.

In a big bowl, place the asparagus, add olive oil to the top, and toss to coat.

Add to the bowl the syrup, paprika, pepper, and salt and toss to coat.

In a medium, shallow bowl, mix the almond meal and nutritional yeast.

Line a cookie sheet with parchment paper and set to the side

Individually add each asparagus piece to the bowl, coating with your crumb mixture.

Place the asparagus on a lined cookie sheet; be sure not to overlap them.

Bake for 20 minutes or until brown.

Remove from the oven and serve.

Chocolate Fudge

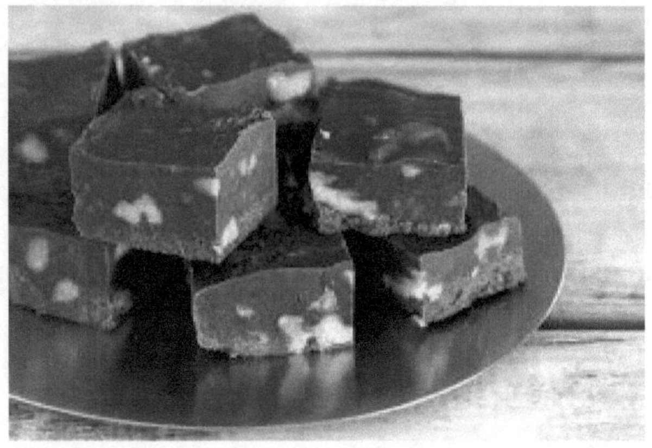

Preparation time: 10 minutes

Servings: 12

Ingredients:

4 oz unsweetened dark chocolate

3/4 cup coconut butter

15 drops liquid stevia

1 tsp vanilla extract

Directions:

Melt coconut butter and dark chocolate.

Add ingredients to the large bowl and combine well.

Pour mixture into a silicone loaf pan and place in refrigerator until set.

Cut into pieces and serve.

Coconut Peanut Butter Fudge

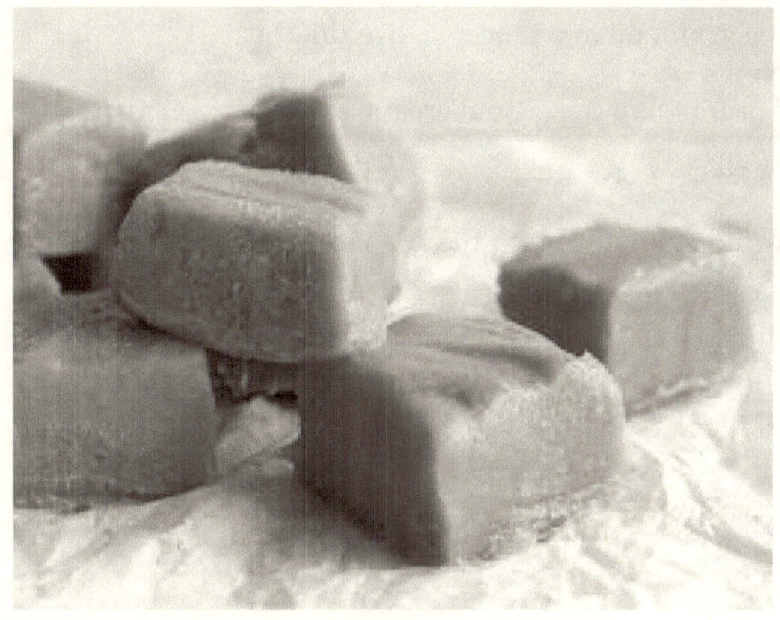

Preparation time: 1 hour 15 minutes

Servings: 20

Ingredients:

12 oz smooth peanut butter

3 tbsp coconut oil

4 tbsp coconut cream

15 drops liquid stevia

Pinch of salt

Directions:

Line baking tray with parchment paper.

Melt coconut oil in a saucepan over low heat.

Add peanut butter, coconut cream, stevia, and salt in a saucepan. Stir well.

Pour fudge mixture into the prepared baking tray and place in refrigerator for 1 hour.

Cut into pieces and serve.

Raspberry Chia Pudding

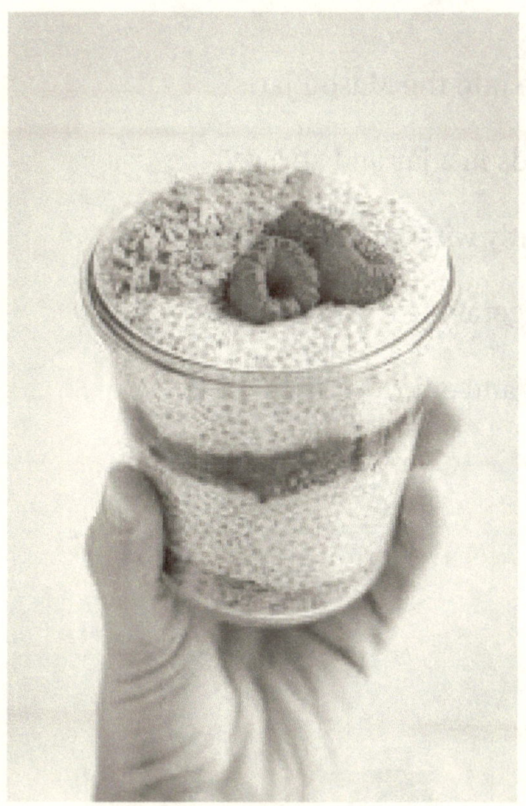

Preparation time: 3 hours 10 minutes

Servings: 2

Ingredients:

4 tbsp chia seeds

1 cup coconut milk

1/2 cup raspberries

Directions:

Add raspberry and coconut milk in a blender and blend until smooth.

Pour mixture into the Mason jar.

Add chia seeds in a jar and stir well.

Close jar tightly with lid and shake well.

Place in refrigerator for 3 hours.

Serve chilled and enjoy.

Chocolate Fat Bomb

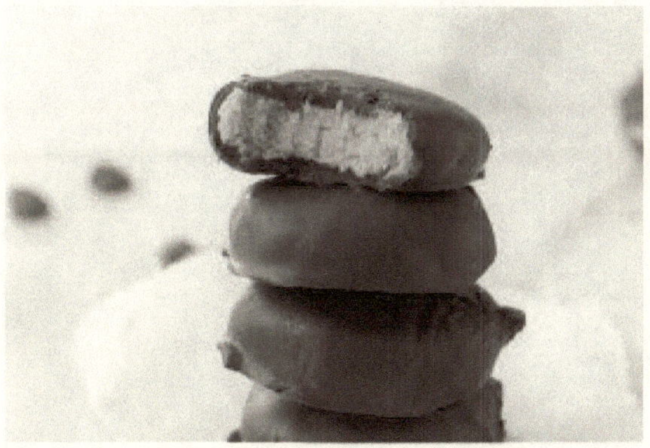

Preparation time: 5 min.

Servings: 14

Ingredients:

1 tbsp. liquid sweetener of your choice.

¼ c. of the following:

coconut oil, melted

cocoa powder

½ c. almond butter

Direction:

Mix the ingredients in a medium bowl until smooth. Pour into the candy molds or ice cube trays.

Put in the freezer to set.

Store in freezer.

Vanilla Cheesecake

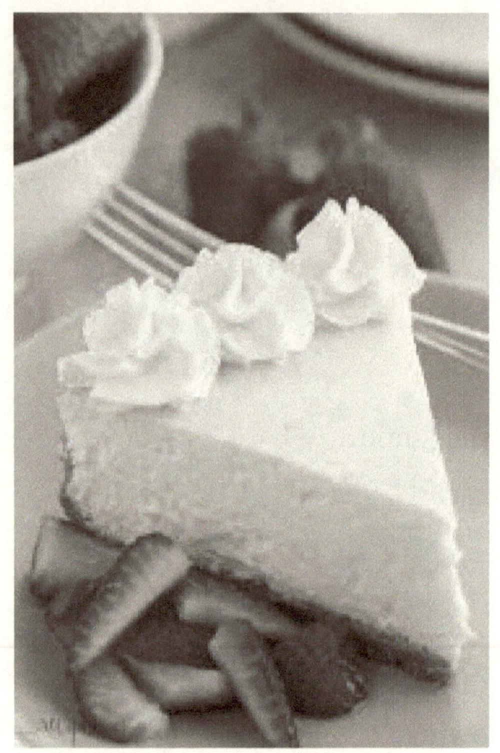

Preparation time: 3 hr. 20 min.

Servings: 10

Ingredients:

1 tbsp. vanilla extract,

2 ½ tbsp. lemon juice

½ c. coconut oil

1/8 t. stevia powder

6 tbsp. coconut milk

1 ½ c. blanched almonds soaked

Crust:

2 tbsp. coconut oil

1 ½ c. almonds

Direction:

For the Crust:

1. In a food processor, add the almonds and coconut oil and pulse until crumbles start to form.

2. Line a 7-inch springform pan with parchment paper and firmly press the crust into the bottom.

For the Sauce:

3. Bring a saucepan of water to a boil and soak the almonds for 2 hours. Drain and shake to dry.

4. Next, add the almonds to the food processor and blend until completely smooth.

5. Add vanilla, lemon, coconut oil, stevia, and coconut milk and blend until smooth.

6. Pour over the crust and freeze overnight or for a minimum of 3 hours.

7. Serve and enjoy.

Chocolate Mousse

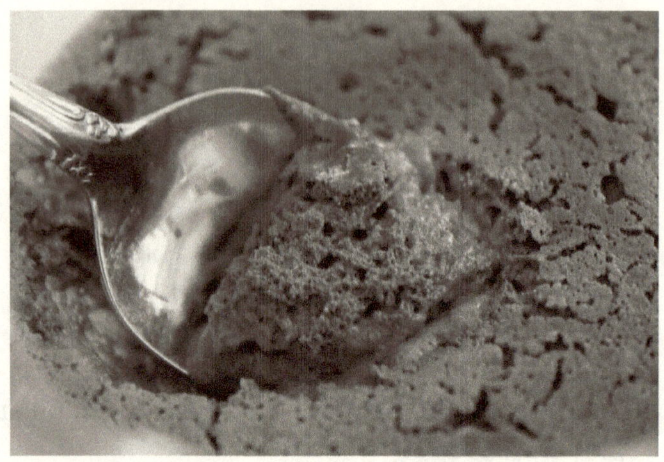

Preparation time: 5 min.

Servings: 2

Ingredients:

6 drops liquid stevia extract

½ t. cinnamon

3 tbsp. cocoa powder, unsweetened

1 c. coconut milk

Direction:

On the day before, place the coconut milk into the refrigerator overnight.

Remove the coconut milk from the refrigerator; it should be very thick.

Whisk in cocoa powder with an electric mixer.

Add stevia and cinnamon and whip until combined.

Place in individual bowls and serve and enjoy.

Avocado Chocolate Mousse

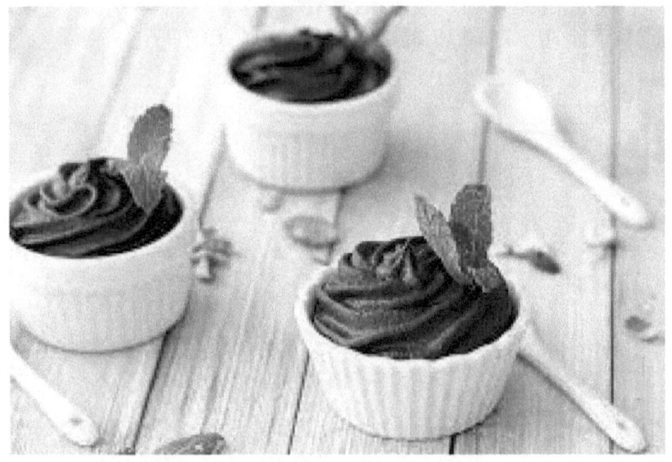

Preparation time: 3 hr. 20 min.

Servings: 4

Ingredients:

2 pinches sea salt

4 tbsp. sweetener of your choice

1 c. almond milk, unsweetened

2 avocados, peeled and pitted

Direction:

Blend everything using a machine of your choice, as long as the consistency becomes smooth for a mousse. If too thick, add some more coconut milk, ¼ teaspoon at a time.

Serve and enjoy.

Coconut Fat Bombs

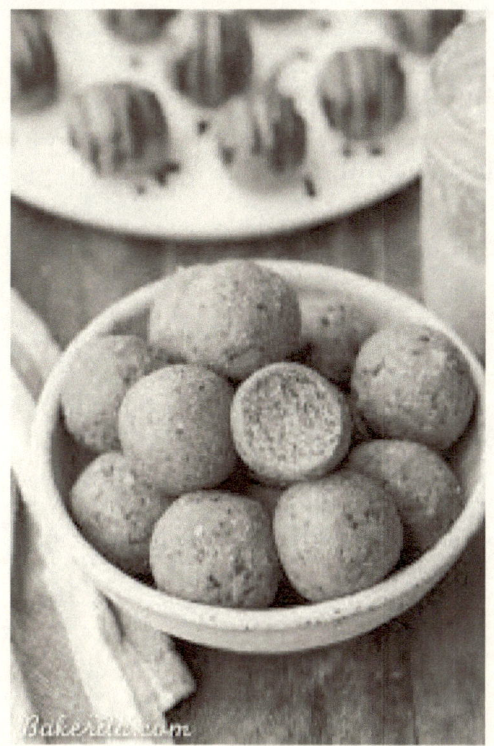

Preparation time: 1 hr. 5 min.

Servings: 4

Ingredients:

20 drops liquid stevia

1 c. coconut flakes, unsweetened

¾ c. coconut oil

1 can coconut milk

Direction:

In a big microwave-safe mixing bowl, add coconut oil and warm on low power for 20 seconds to melt.

Whisk in coconut milk and stevia into the oil.

Add coconut flakes; combine well.

Pour into candy molds or ice cube trays and freeze for 1 hour.

Serve and enjoy.

Coconut Cupcakes

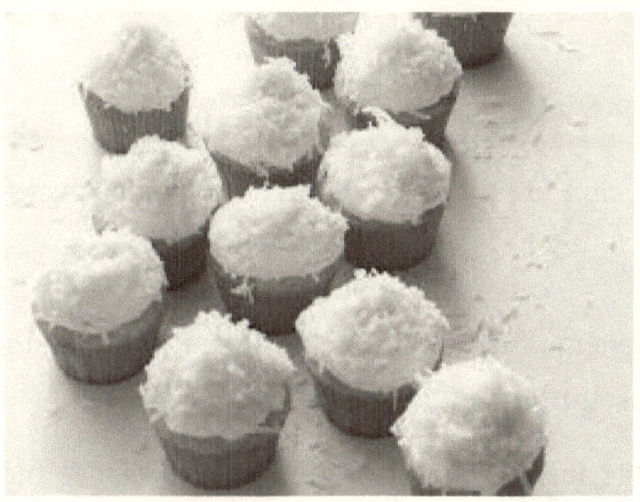

Preparation time: 1 hr. 5 min.

Servings: 18

Ingredients:

1 tbsp. vanilla

1 t. baking soda

1 c. erythritol

4 t. baking powder

1 ¼ c. coconut milk

¾ c. coconut flour

14 tbsp. arrowroot powder

2 c. almond meal

½ c. coconut oil

Whipped Cream:

1 t. vanilla

¼ c. erythritol

2 13.5 oz. cans full-fat coconut milk, refrigerated overnight

Direction:

1. Prepare a muffin tin with muffin liners and bring the oven to 350 heat setting.

2. In a big mixing bowl, add all the ingredients and beat on medium-high speed until it turns to a batter-like consistency. If too dry, add ¼ teaspoon of water at a time.

3. Fill the cupcake cups with the batter, three-quarters full.

4. Bake for 20 minutes or until the cupcakes are firm.

5. Place in the refrigerator to cool.

6. While cupcakes are cooling, make the whipped cream.

7. Remove the coconut milk from the fridge and pour the clear coconut water from the milk.

8. In a big mixing bowl, add the vanilla and erythritol; beat until fluffy.

9. Ice the cupcakes and serve.

10. Serve and enjoy.

Pumpkin Truffles

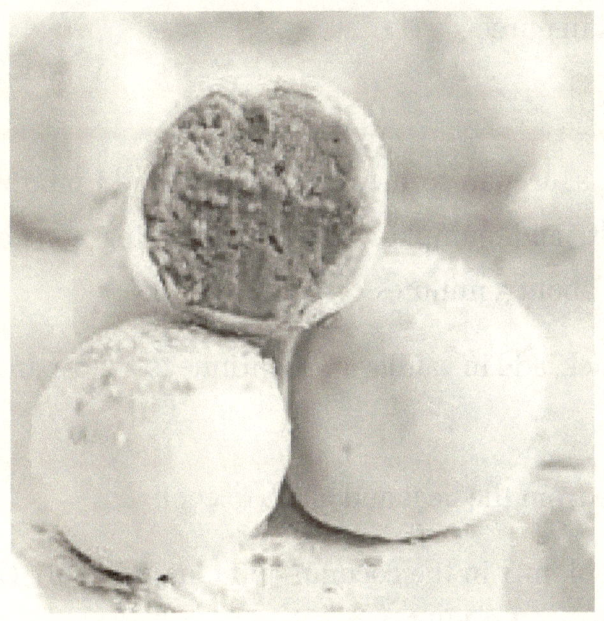

Preparation time: 15 min.

Servings: 12

Ingredients:

1 t. cinnamon

2 tbsp. coconut sugar

3 tbsp. coconut flour

½ c. almond flour

1 t. pumpkin pie spice

¼ t. salt

½ t. vanilla extract

¼ c. maple syrup

1 c. pumpkin puree

Direction:

1. Bring a saucepan to medium heat and add pumpkin puree, syrup, salt, and pumpkin pie spice, stirring constantly until thickened about 5 minutes.

2. Once thick, add in vanilla and continue to stir for an additional minute.

3. Remove from the heat and allow to cool.

4. Once cool, mix in the coconut and almond flour. Then put in the refrigerator to chill for 10 minutes.

5. Remove from the fridge and mix again. If the dough is too sticky, add in 1 tablespoon of almond flour until you can form a ball with the dough.

6. Form 12 balls using your hands with the dough.

7. In a little bowl, combine coconut sugar and cinnamon.

8. Roll each ball into the cinnamon-sugar mixture.

9. Serve and enjoy.

Raspberry Truffles

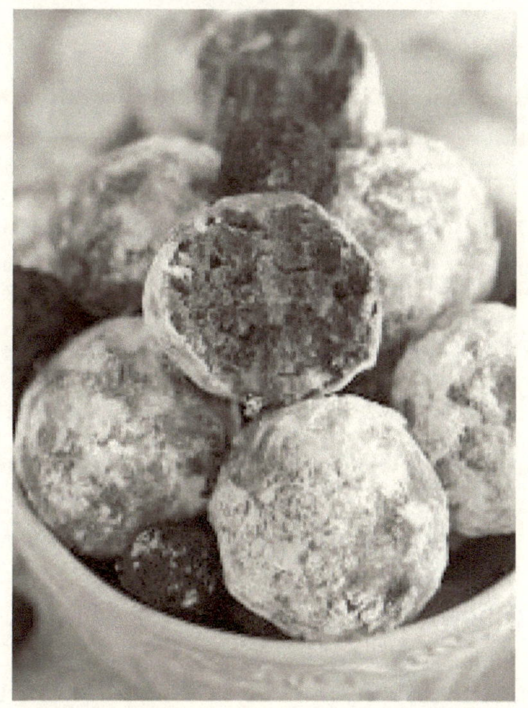

Preparation time: 15 min.

Servings: 36

Ingredients:

2 tbsp. cocoa powder, unsweetened

6 oz. of the following:

fresh raspberries, dry

chocolate, bittersweet, finely chopped

coconut milk, full-fat

Direction:

1. Prepare a cookie sheet with parchment paper and set to the side.

2. Warm a saucepan over medium heat, and add coconut milk.

3. Remove from the heat and add the chocolate with a rubber spatula, stirring to melt the chocolate 4. Once smooth, add the raspberries, 5-8 at a time. Stir to coat.

5. Using two forks, remove the raspberries from the chocolate sauce, allowing the excess sauce to drop back into the pan. Repeat this step until you have coated all raspberries.

6. Place the raspberries in the refrigerator for 1 hour or until firm.

7. In a shallow bowl with a lid, add the cocoa powder.

8. Once truffles are firm, place 5 to 8 truffles in the bowl and shake to coat with cocoa powder.

9. Return to the refrigerator until ready to serve.

Strawberry Ice Cream

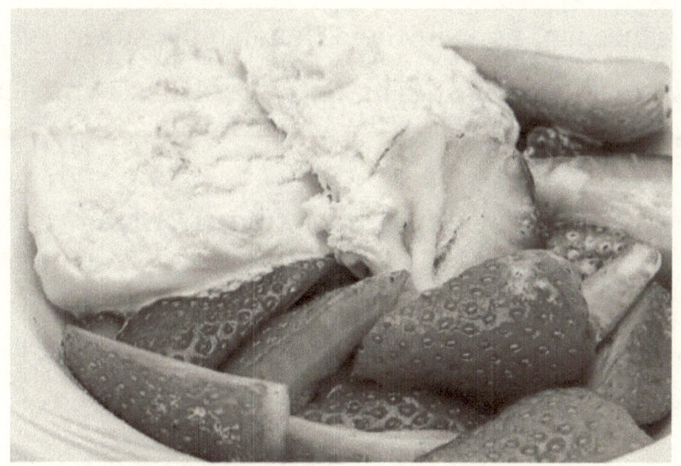

Preparation time: 7 hr. 60 min.

Servings: 8

Ingredients:

½ t. salt

1 tbsp. strawberry extract

1 c. strawberry puree

¼ c. maple syrup

½ c. sweetener of your choice

14 oz. coconut milk

14 oz. coconut cream

You will need an ice cream maker for this recipe.

Direction:

1. Place your ice cream bowl in the freezer one day before.

2. In a saucepan, pour in the coconut milk, sugar, syrup, and coconut cream, gently stirring until it reaches a simmer. Then remove from the heat.

3. Add in salt, strawberry extract, and strawberry puree then blend with an immersion blender until smooth.

4. Transfer the mixture into a container with a lid and place in the freezer to chill for 30 minutes.

5. Following the directions on your ice cream maker, churn the mixture for about 20-40 minutes until a soft-serve consistency is reached.

6. Transfer to a loaf pan and place in the freezer for approximately 6 hours.

7. Scoop and serve.

Quick Chocó Brownie

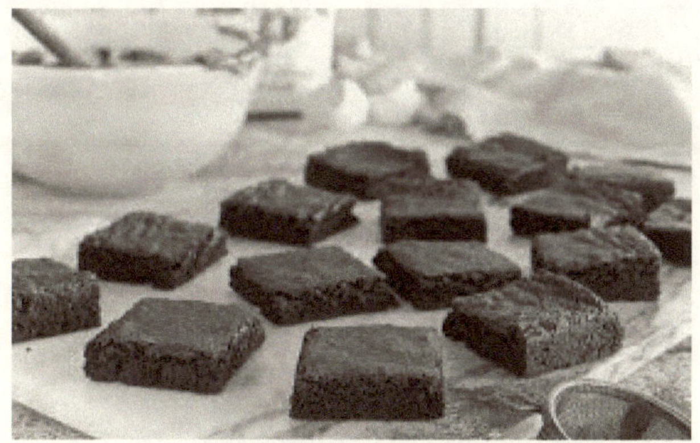

Preparation time: 10 minutes

Servings: 1

Ingredients:

1/4 cup almond milk

1 tbsp cocoa powder

1 scoop chocolate protein powder

1/2 tsp baking powder

Directions:

In a microwave-safe mug blend together baking powder, protein powder, and cocoa.

Add almond milk in a mug and stir well.

Place mug in microwave and microwave for 30 seconds.

Serve and enjoy.

Chocó Chia Pudding

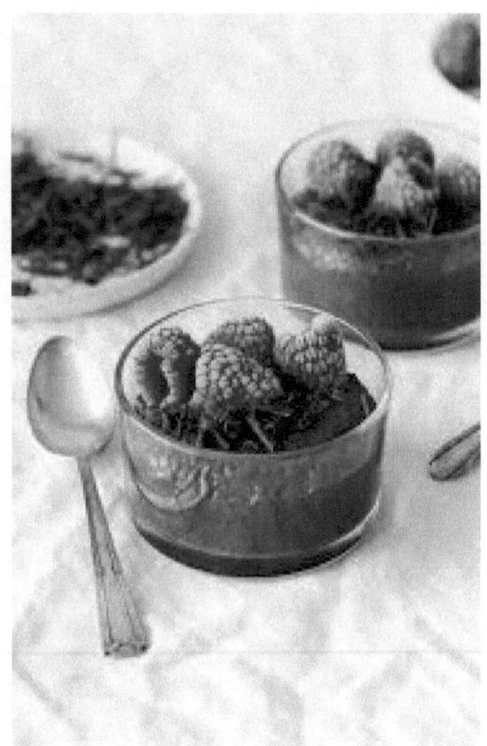

Preparation time: 10 minutes

Servings: 6

Ingredients:

2 1/2 cups coconut milk

2 scoops stevia extract powder

6 tbsp cocoa powder

1/2 cup chia seeds

1/2 tsp vanilla extract

1/8 cup xylitol

1/8 tsp salt

Directions:

Add all ingredients into the blender and blend until smooth.

Pour mixture into the glass container and place in refrigerator.

Serve chilled and enjoy.

Smooth Chocolate Mousse

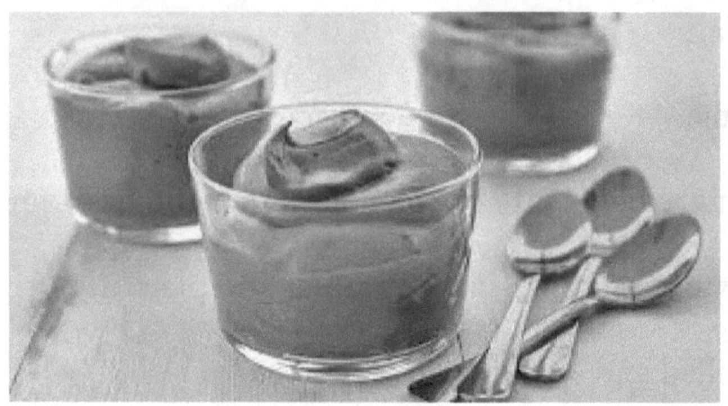

Preparation time: 10 minutes

Servings: 2

Ingredients:

1/2 tsp cinnamon

3 tbsp unsweetened cocoa powder

1 cup creamed coconut milk

10 drops liquid stevia

Directions:

Place coconut milk can in the refrigerator for overnight; it should get thick and the solids separate from water.

Transfer thick part into the large mixing bowl without water.

Add remaining ingredients to the bowl and whip with electric mixer until smooth.

Serve and enjoy.

Quick Chocó Brownie

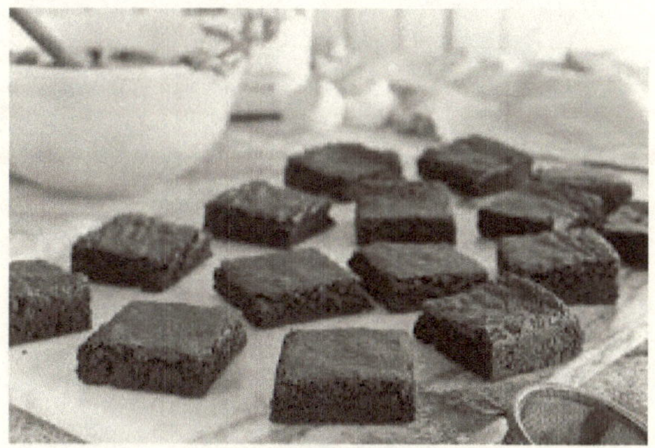

Preparation time: 10 minutes

Servings: 1

Ingredients:

1/4 cup almond milk

1 tbsp cocoa powder

1 scoop chocolate protein powder

1/2 tsp baking pow der

Directions:

In a microwave-safe mug blend together baking powder, protein powder, and cocoa.

Add almond milk in a mug and stir well.

Place mug in microwave and microwave for 30 seconds.

Serve and enjoy.

Chocó Chia Pudding

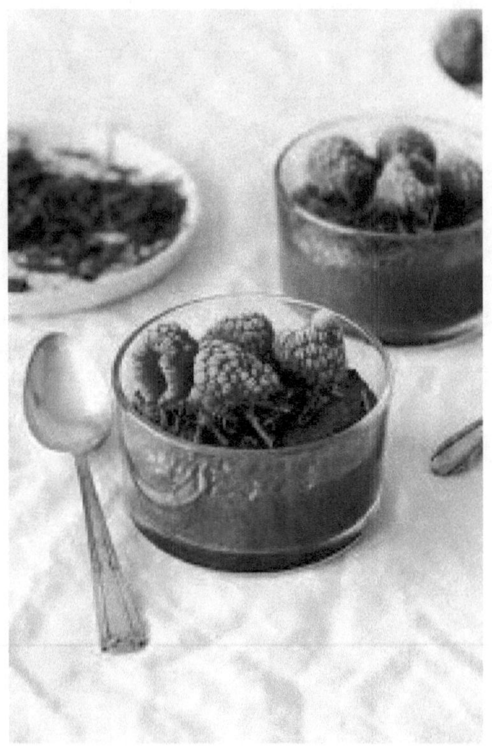

Preparation time: 10 minutes

Servings: 6

Ingredients:

2 1/2 cups coconut milk

2 scoops stevia extract powder

6 tbsp cocoa powder

1/2 cup chia seeds

1/2 tsp vanilla extract

1/8 cup xylitol

1/8 tsp salt

Directions:

Add all ingredients into the blender and blend until smooth.

Pour mixture into the glass container and place in refrigerator.

Serve chilled and enjoy.

Smooth Chocolate Mousse

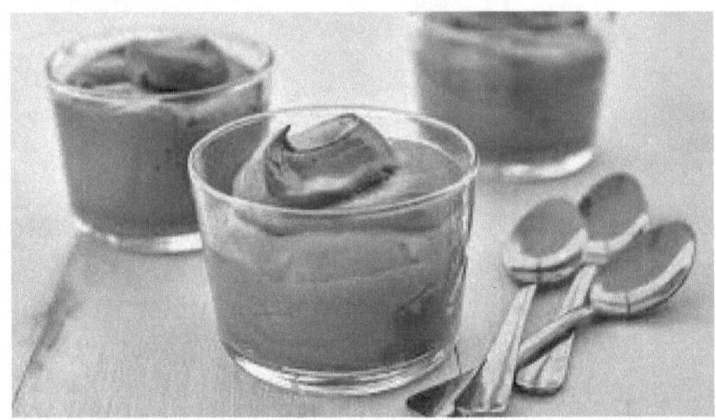

Preparation time: 10 minutes

Servings: 2

Ingredients:

1/2 tsp cinnamon

3 tbsp unsweetened cocoa powder

1 cup creamed coconut milk

10 drops liquid stevia

Directions:

Place coconut milk can in the refrigerator for overnight; it should get thick and the solids separate from water.

Transfer thick part into the large mixing bowl without water.

Add remaining ingredients to the bowl and whip with electric mixer until smooth.

Serve and enjoy.

Fatty Chocolate Bombs

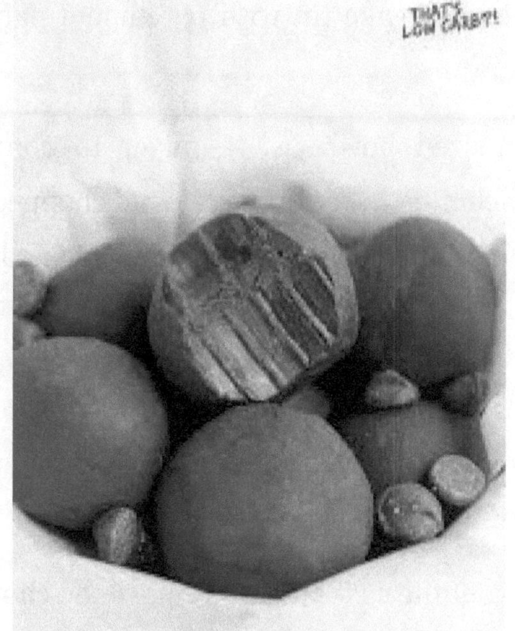

Preparation time: 40 minutes

Servings: 12

Ingredients:

¼ cup organic soy protein, chocolate fl avor

½ cup coconut butter

¼ cup coconut oil

½ tsp. stevia powder

pinch of salt

a few fresh mint leaves

Direction

Line a small square cake tin with parchment paper and set it aside.

In a medium-sized bowl, use a mixer to combine all the ingredients, including the optional salt and chopped mint leaves. Make sure all ingredients are incorporated and no lumps remain in the batter.

Pour the mixture into the prepared tin.

Transfer the cake tin to the freezer and allow the mixture to set for about 30 minutes.

Once set, take out the cake tin and remove the chocolate chunk. Cut it into 12 squares.

Serve the fatty chocolate bombs with more optional mint leaves on top and enjoy!

Peanut Butter Bombs

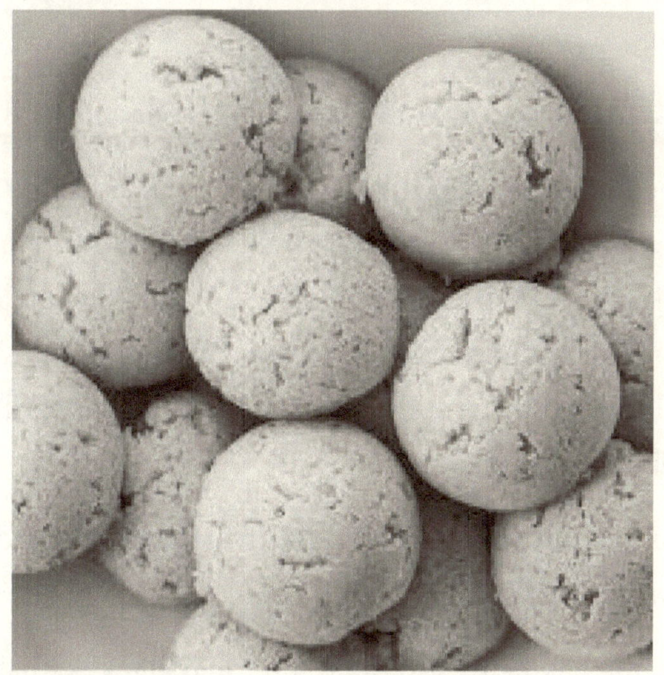

Preparation time: 40 minutes

Servings: 20

Ingredients:

1 cup peanut butter

6 tbsp. coconut flour

¼ cup low-carb maple syrup

¼ cup organic soy protein, chocolate flavor

pinch of salt

1 tbsp. water

¾ cup dark chocolate, 85% cocoa or higher, crushed

Direction

Line a large baking tray with parchment paper and set it aside.

In a medium-sized bowl, use a mixer to combine all the ingredients except the crushed dark chocolate. If desired, add the optional pinch of salt. Make sure all ingredients are well incorporated and no lumps remain in the batter. Add the optional water if the mixture is too thick – the batter should be spreadable.

Use your hands to form 20 balls and divide these over the surface of the baking tray.

Transfer the baking tray to the freezer and allow the balls to set for about 15 minutes.

Fill a small saucepan with water and put it over medium heat. Place a smaller, heat-resistant metal bowl in the water and put the crushed chocolate into it.

Melt the chocolate au bain-marie (in the bowl) and leave the container in the water. Be careful to keep any water from getting in the chocolate. Make sure the chocolate doesn't boil because it will ruin the flavor.

Take the peanut butter bombs from the freezer and roll each ball in the molten chocolate, using two forks to help you. Put each ball back onto the tray and allow the molten chocolate to firm up. Repeat this step for every peanut butter bomb.

Refrigerate the bombs for 15 minutes, until the chocolate layer is completely firm.

Serve the peanut butter bombs and enjoy!

Cheesecake Cups

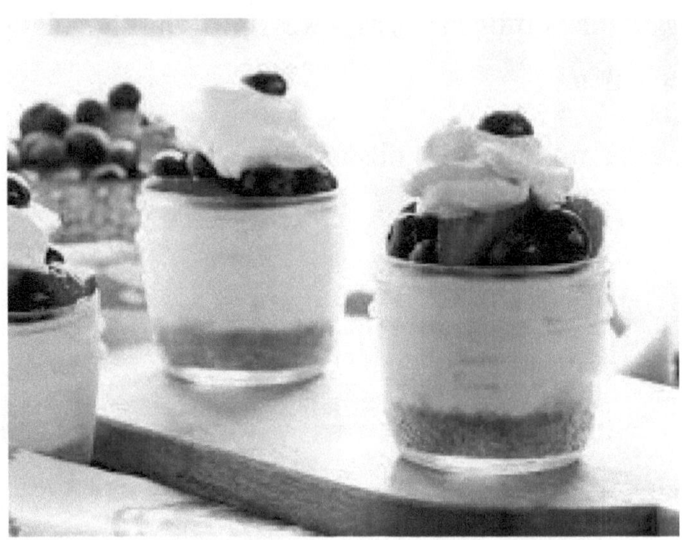

Preparation time: 10 minutes

Cooking time: 4 minutes

Servings: 12

Ingredients: Crust:

½ cup pumpkin seeds, r aw

6 tbsp. shredded coconut, unsweetened

3 tbsp. coconut oil

2 tbsp. organic soy protein, vanilla flavor

½ tsp. stevia powder

Pinch of salt

Filling:

6 tbsp. coconut oil

6 tbsp. almond butter

6 tbsp. coconut cream

2 tbsp. lemon juice

2 tbsp. organic soy protein, vanilla flavor

Pinch of salt

¼ tsp. xanthan gum

¼ tsp. stevia powder

Direction

Line a cupcake tin with 6 cupcake liners.

Heat a small frying pan over medium-high heat.

Toast the pumpkin seeds in the frying pan, stirring occasionally for about 4 minutes.

Add the shredded coconut and stir thoroughly to toast everything evenly.

Take the frying pan off the heat and allow the ingredients to cool down before transferring them into a food processor or blender. Pulse the pumpkin seeds and shredded coconut into small crumbs.

Transfer the crumbs to a medium-sized bowl and add the remaining crust ingredients.

Combine all ingredients into a thick dough and divide this mixture into six equal-sized balls.

Put one ball into each of the cupcake liners, pressing and flattening the balls into a crust at the bottom of each cupcake liner.

Transfer the tin into the freezer and prepare the filling.

Heat a medium-sized saucepan over medium heat and add the coconut oil. Remove the saucepan from the heat once the coconut oil has melted.

Put the melted coconut oil, almond butter, coconut cream, lemon juice, organic soy protein, and a pinch of salt to the (uncleaned) food processor or blender. Process these ingredients until well combined with a smooth and creamy texture.

Add the optional xanthan gum and stevia. Xanthan gum will help thicken the cheesecake fat bombs, while the stevia will add a sweeter flavor. Use slightly more or less stevia to taste.

Take the cupcake tin out of the freezer and top all crusts with filling. Make sure to divide the filling equally among the 6 cups with a tablespoon.

Transfer the tin back into the fridge until the cups are firm.

Serve the cheesecake cups at room temperature and enjoy!

Cashew Cocoa Bombs

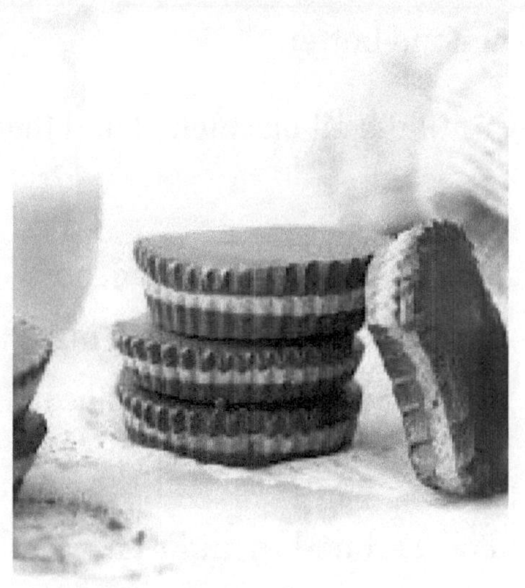

Preparation time: 30 minutes

Servings: 10

Ingredients:

1 cup coconut oil

1 cup almond butter

¼ cup coconut flou r

¼ cup cocoa powder

¼ cup organic soy protein, chocolate flavor

Pinch of salt

1 cup raw cashews, unsalted

Direction

Heat a medium-sized saucepan over medium heat and add the coconut oil and almond butter.

Stir occasionally until the oil has melted and the ingredients are combined.

Pour the mixture into a medium-sized bowl and, while the mixture is still warm, stir in the remaining ingredients except the cashews. Make sure all ingredients are well combined.

Transfer the bowl into the freezer until the dough has become firm. This should take around 15 minutes.

Crush the cashews into small pieces by using a coffee grinder, food processor, or blender. Spread the crushed cashew bits over a large plate.

Make sure that the dough is firm before making the fat bombs.

Take 1 tablespoon of the firm dough mixture and roll it into a ball. Roll the ball in the crushed cashews and transfer it onto a baking tray or plate. Repeat this step for all 10 balls.

Put the baking tray in the fridge for a few minutes to allow the bombs to firm up.

Take the tray out of the fridge, serve the cashew cocoa bombs and enjoy!

Cinnamon-Vanilla Bites

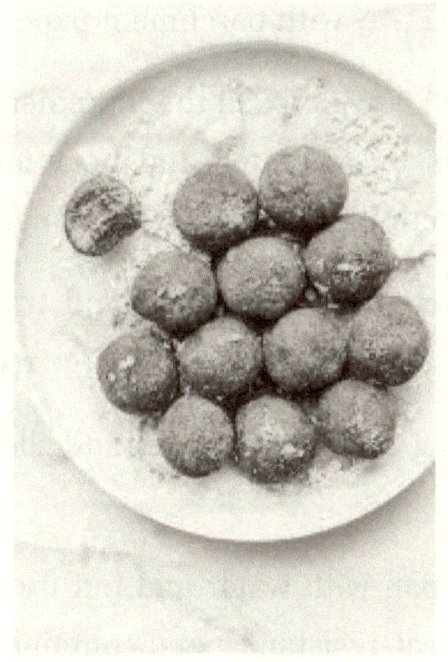

Preparation time: 40 minutes

Servings: 20

Ingredients:

1 cup coconut oil

1 cup cocoa butter

6 tbsp. almond butter

2 tsp. cinnamon

1 tsp. vanilla extract

¼ cup organic soy protein, vanilla flavor

2 tbsp. water

½ cup dark chocolate

Direction

Line a large baking tray with parchment paper and set it aside.

In a medium-sized bowl, mix all the ingredients together. Make sure everything is incorporated and no lumps remain in the dough. Add some additional water if the dough is too thick.

Make sure the dough is spreadable and transfer it onto the baking tray. Spread the mixture into a large rectangular chunk.

Transfer the baking tray to the freezer and allow to set for about 15 minutes.

Fill a small saucepan with water and put it over medium heat. Place a smaller, heat-resistant metal container inside the water and put the crushed chocolate into it.

Melt the chocolate au bain-marie (in the bowl in the water). Be careful to keep any water from getting in the chocolate. Make sure the chocolate doesn't boil because it will ruin the flavor.

Take the baking tray out of the freezer and cut the dough into 10 or 20 squares.

Using a fork, dip each square into the molten chocolate. Repeat this for all the cinnamon-vanilla bites, putting each one back onto the baking tray.

Refrigerate the squares for abou t 15 minutes, until the chocolate coating has firmed up. Serve and enjoy!

Chapter 9: 4 Weeks Meal Plan

DAYS	BREAKFAST	LUNCH/DINNER	SNACKS/DESSERT
1	Avocado with halloumi cheese	Herb Spaghetti Squash	Lemon Mousse
2	Vegetarian pizza recipe	Delicious Cabbage Steaks	Avocado Pudding
3	Spinach lasagne with zucchini	Mexican Cauliflower Rice	Almond Butter Brownies
4	Keto rice with cheddar cheese	Asparagus Mash	Simple Almond Butter Fudge
5	Caprese	Creamy Squash Soup	Crispy Squash Chips
6	Wege pasta	Spinach with Coconut Milk	Paprika Nuts

7	Microwave Quick Keto Bread	Sautéed Brussels sprouts	Basil Zoodles and Olives
8	Shakshuka with goat cheese	Turnip Carrot Salad	Roasted Beetroot Noodles
9	Low Carb Chocolate Muffins	Baked Asparagus	Turnip Fries
10	Coconut flour biscuits with cheese	Avocado Mint Soup	Lime and Chili Carrots Noodles
11	Breakfast in a cup with ham and cheese	Vegetable Salad	Cinnamon Granola
12	Coconut flour biscuits with cheese	Lemon Zucchini Noodles	Chocolate Granola
13	Aerial keto waffles	Classic Cabbage Slaw	Radish Chips

14	Keto omelet with minced meat	Delicious Herb Cauliflower Rice	Asparagus Fries
15	Peanut Butter Pancakes	Mushroom Asparagus	Chocolate Fudge
16	Tuna Egg Rolls	Tomato Eggplant Spinach Salad	Coconut Peanut Butter Fudge
17	Waffle Chicken Sandwich	Roasted Cauliflower	Raspberry Chia Pudding
18	Carrot Cream Muffins	Cauliflower Coconut Rice	Chocolate Fat Bomb
19	Chia Seed Pumpkin Pudding	Ginger Avocado Kale Salad	Vanilla Cheesecake
20	Matcha Chia Seed Pudding	Refreshing Cucumber Salad	Chocolate Mousse
21	Pepperoni Cheese Muffins	Truffle Parmesan Salad	Avocado Chocolate Mousse

22	Cheese and Egg Tart	Cashew Siam Salad	Coconut Fat Bombs
23	Low carb muesli	Avocado and Cauliflower Hummus	Coconut Cupcakes
24	Garlic Cauliflower Fried Rice	Raw Zoodles with Avocado 'N Nuts	Pumpkin Truffles
25	Bacon Egg Muffins	Cauliflower Sushi	Raspberry Truffles
26	Coconut flour biscuits with cheese	Spinach and Mashed Tofu Salad	Strawberry Ice Cream
27	Vegetarian pizza recipe	Keto Curry Almond Bread	Smooth Chocolate Mousse
28	Spinach lasagne with zucchini	Egg Roll Bowl	Coconut Peanut Butter Fudge

Conclusion

We have come to the end of this book and you are likely wondering if this diet is right for you. Answer this: Are you looking for a diet that is proven safe and effective?

The Ketogenic Vegan diet is very beneficial for your health and stamina. The combination of these two diets is one of the best you can find for your physical well-being and mental performance. Commit to it and you will reap the benefits!

Remember, that your diet plan is more than a way for you to lose weight and present yourself as an appealing tidbit to outsiders. It is about you, your health, your choices, and how you choose to be – it is, in short, about how you allow them to see you. Which is why it is so important that you choose a diet plan that works for you, based on your lifestyle and your cultural and social habits.